THE NATURAL WAY SERIES

Increasing numbers of people worldwide are falling victim to illnesses which modern medicine, for all its technical advances, often seems powerless to prevent – and sometimes actually causes. To find cures for these so-called 'diseases of civilization' more and more people are turning to 'natural' medicine for an answer. *The Natural Way* series aims to offer clear, practical and reliable guidance to the safest, gentlest and most effective treatments available – and so to give sufferers and their families the information they need to make their own choices about the most suitable treatments.

Other titles in the Natural Way *series*

THE NATURAL WAY WITH

Heart Disease

Richard Thomas

Approved by the
**AMERICAN HOLISTIC MEDICAL ASSOCIATION
& BRITISH HOLISTIC MEDICAL ASSOCIATION**

Series medical consultants
Dr Peter Albright MD & Dr David Peters MD

Series editor
Richard Thomas

ELEMENT
Shaftesbury, Dorset ● Rockport, Massachusetts
Brisbane, Queensland

© Richard Thomas 1994

First published in Great Britain in 1994 by
Element Books Limited
Shaftesbury, Dorset SP7 8BP

Published in the USA in 1994 by
Element Books, Inc.
PO Box 830, Rockport, MA 01966

Published in Australia in 1994 by
Element Books Limited for
Jacaranda Wiley Limited
33 Park Road, Milton, Brisbane 4064

Reprinted 1995

Cover design by Max Fairbrother
Designed and typeset by Linda Reed and Joss Nizan
Printed and bound in Great Britain by
BPC Paperbacks Limited

British Library Cataloguing in Publication
data available

Library of Congress Cataloging in Publication Data
Thomas, Richard. 1943-
The natural way with heart disease/Richard Thomas.
Includes bibliographical references and index.
1. Heart–Diseases–Alternative treatment.
I. Title. II. Series.
RC684.A48T46 1994
616.1'206–dc20   94–13149

ISBN 1–85230–494–4

For my parents,
two of the most genuinely 'good-hearted' people
it has been my privilege to know

———————————

Contents

Acknowledgements

Thanks for help and support to Dr Peter Albright and the American Holistic Medical Association, Dr David Peters and the British Holistic Medical Association, Lord Colwyn and the Arterial Health Foundation, Richard F Brown and the UK Arterial Disease Clinics, Dr Wayne Perry, Dr Peter Nixon, Dr Stephen Davies, Dr Richard Passwater, Dr Linus Pauling, Dr Tamara Voronina, Harald Gaier and the International Federation of Practitioners of Natural Therapeutics, Patrick Holford and the Institute of Optimum Nutrition, John Stirling and Biocare UK Ltd, Rhaya Jordan and Blackmores UK Ltd, Cheryl Thallon and Solgar Vitamins UK Ltd, John Redman and Lamberts Healthcare Ltd, Howard Kent and the Yoga for Health Foundation, the Association of British Pharmaceutical Industries, Association of Medical Research Charities, British Heart Foundation, Department of Health, European Aspirin Foundation, Medical Research Council, National Blood Authority, Research Council for Complementary Medicine, Royal Society of Medicine, National Sports Medical Institute, Nicola, Alexander, Carol, Craig and Paul – and last but not, of course, least to everyone at Element Books in both Britain and America and for their faith, enthusiasm and understanding, especially to Michael, David, Annie, Julia, Roger Skye and Del.

Foreword

by Lord Colwyn
President of the Arterial Health Foundation

Every day someone somewhere in the Western world is being told by doctors to go home and wait patiently for the inevitable. They have such severe heart disease they are being told there is nothing further conventional medicine can do for them. For a long time this attitude has troubled me. The simple fact is that there are genuine alternatives available for the treatment of coronary artery disease but most doctors will have little to do with them. As with most conditions, including those as severe as heart disease and cancer, they seem to be locked into an almost conditioned response reflecting the assumptions of past training, seemingly allowing little or no room for imaginative, innovative and flexible new thinking.

Heart disease is one area in which I would have thought, and hoped, new ideas would have been enthusiastically welcomed. As most people know, it is the single biggest killer in the 'developed' world, and the statistics suggest the problem is not getting any better. Indeed, with an increasingly ageing population in areas like Europe and North America, this is hardly surprising.

In Britain, where I try to play an active part in health

and medical politics and where there is one of the worst
records of heart disease in the world, the government
has set out a policy to try to reduce heart deaths by 40
per cent by the year 2000. But rather than cast far and
wide for solutions the standard medical response has
been to call for an increase in the textbook treatments of
surgery and drug therapy – even when those same
treatments have been amply demonstrated, particularly
in North America, to be not only over-used and
extremely costly but also dangerous, traumatic and
short-term. They are not even a cure.

The idea, therefore, of promoting prevention before
intervention and of setting out the benefits of gentle
treatments before the relative trauma of surgery and
side-effects of powerful drugs seems to me to be
eminently sensible and logical and worthy of the
greatest support. That is why I am delighted to write the
foreword to the first in this excellent new series of books.
If ever there was an idea whose time has come this is it
and I wish it, and those who stand to benefit by reading
it, the success it and they both deserve.

The Lord Colwyn CBE, BDS, LDSRCS
President
The Arterial Health Foundation
London, UK

January 1994

Introduction

Heart disease is the single biggest cause of death in the Western world. In America and Britain, for example, it kills as many people as all other diseases put together, including cancer. Everyone in the Western world dies with (though not necessarily, of course, of) heart disease; we start to develop it almost from birth. Most people reading this are likely to have heart disease. Nearly half will die of it or related problems such as stroke. These days an increasing number of quite young people, even children in their teens, have advanced heart disease.

Heart disease is a problem of pandemic proportions in the so-called developed world, affecting not just sufferers but also family, friends, work colleagues, healthcarers and administrators on whom its effects can be just as devastating. Literally billions are spent on its treatment worldwide (more than £3 billion a year by the USA, Japan, Britain, Germany and Switzerland alone).

Those are the stark facts. But this book is not a catalogue of doom and gloom. The very opposite in fact. It's central message is one of hope, that there is an answer. Though devastating, heart disease is thoroughly researched and well understood. It is also largely preventable. The main argument revolves not so much around what causes it or even how to avoid it but how best to treat it. Orthodox medicine has opted largely for the 'big guns' of drugs and surgery and, until relatively recently, has tended to ignore softer, gentler alternatives – even as an intermediate stage in care. If you show signs of heart disease, such as angina, the typical response is often to want to rush you in for a bypass operation. As many specialists now concede, you may not need surgery at all and may be better doing something as simple, for example, as changing your diet, taking some exercise and learning relaxation techniques to reduce and manage stress levels.

This book is intended to introduce you to those softer, gentler, safer alternatives. It aims to be above all practical. The natural way with heart disease is prevention first and foremost, but failing that it is seeking treatment that does not involve either taking drugs or having surgery. But this book is not concerned with attacking any one system. It is interested most of all in opening doors, in helping you get the best answers there are so that you can make an informed choice about what might be the best treatment for you, and get it.

Since heart and arteries are intimately connected doctors use terms like coronary artery disease (CAD), coronary heart disease (CHD), cardiovascular disease (CVD) and ischaemic heart disease (IHD) when they talk about the problem. In this book we describe all these conditions simply as 'heart disease'. Our aim is to show you how to avoid heart disease, how to recognize if you have it, how to check if you have it and what to do about it if you have – without having to be drugged, cut open or in any other way operated upon, a process known in medical circles as a major intervention. This book aims to show how to avoid a major intervention on your own body if at all possible and therefore how to live as full and active a life as possible without recourse to medical procedures that are drastic, serious and, let's not beat about the bush, downright dangerous. There are better ways and we believe we've found them for you.

Richard Thomas
Burwash
England

January 1994

CHAPTER 1

What is heart disease?

How and why it develops and who it affects

Heart disease does not really exist, at least not in the sense most people understand the word 'disease'. Although we talk about heart disease as if it was caused by something 'out there', attacking the heart directly, this is wrong. A very few unfortunate people are born with heart defects such as 'hole-in-the-heart' or sustain damage to the valves in the heart from rheumatic fever, but for the vast majority heart disease is not something you catch like a 'flu virus.

Heart disease is actually the end result of the gradual deterioration of the network of tubes, including the heart, which supplies blood to the body. Blood should rush round your body like a car round a race-track and in a healthy person this is what happens if your blood vessels are clear and your heart is working properly. It is when blood doesn't flow freely that problems arise.

In fact the heart is usually the innocent party in all this. It is not the first to fail. The main culprits are all those many tubes leading into it and out of it. When, like so much household plumbing, they start to get 'narrow' and 'furred up' the heart is affected and becomes 'sick'. So when we talk about heart disease we really mean 'blood vessel disease'.

At first glance this may not sound too terrible. But the heart is one of the single most important organs in the

body and when it cannot work properly any number of
bodily failures take place, from simple dizziness to
sudden death. Eventually heart disease, if allowed to
develop unchecked, will lead almost inevitably to a
heart attack. A heart attack is simply a heart giving up. It
is so 'creaky' and 'dried up' it cannot work any longer
and so it stops. And when your heart stops you stop.
Your heart is not quite the last thing that stops when you
die but it is the first thing doctors check when someone
collapses and it is the single most important thing they
try to get working again afterwards.

Heart disease, in other words, is the result of having
important blood vessels so clogged up and tense they
are no longer able to let blood flow easily and freely to
the heart – and without that free and easy flow of blood
the heart cannot work.

What causes 'furring up'?

The exact process of what happens is still not fully
understood and experts are even more divided about
what triggers things off in the first place. But what we do
know is that the end result is the build-up of fatty
deposits in blood vessels, and specifically those vessels
called arteries. These deposits are known as *atheromas*
(from a Greek word for 'porridge' to describe their
sticky, gooey-like consistency).

These spongey yellow-coloured deposits start to
accumulate from the moment you are born, and over a
period of time they become hardened or 'calcified'
forming what is called a 'plaque'. Plaques cause both
narrowing and hardening of the arteries – hence two
terms you will hear doctors use to describe the process
of narrowing and hardening of the arteries: *atherosclerosis* and *arteriosclerosis* ('sclerosis' is from another Greek
word meaning hard or tough).

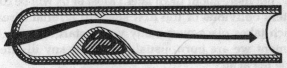

STAGE 1: Diseased artery with deposit

STAGE 2: Surface of deposit breaks exposing raw area

STAGE 3: Blood clot forms and stops circulation

Figure 1 The stages of arterial disease

Atherosclerosis or arteriosclerosis seems to happen in roughly three stages (*see figure 1*):

Stage 1 The 'walls' of the arteries become damaged and worn by the normal process of living in the modern world, especially by the harmful by-products of things we eat, breathe, drink and, yes, worry about or get angry with. (A key element here is the action of particles involved in the normal ageing process called 'free radicals', but more about them later.) Most of us will be completely oblivious of the first stage of arterial disease which takes place over many years, starting from the moment we are born, usually without any ill-effects being felt at all.

Stage 2 Various other fatty chemicals in the blood lodge themselves in these damaged areas, gradually building up and enlarging. These deposits are very unstable and easily break or split as a result of the constant pressure they are under from the bloodstream. Nevertheless this second stage will also not make much of an impact on our general health and well-being until far advanced, usually around middle-age for men but later for women. Many people are never troubled beyond this stage. But unfortunately a large number – around a third of the population of most industrial societies – find themselves victims of the final, and most dangerous, stage: the development of serious heart disease.

Stage 3 With the arteries by now severely restricted, any chance event – such as a piece of plaque breaking off from somewhere else and lodging itself, or a clot of blood covering some damage in an attempt to heal it – can suddenly block the artery and cut off the blood supply completely. Without a proper supply of blood the heart cannot work properly, part or all of it shuts down and has a cramp-like 'seizure' or 'heart attack'.

Warning signs before a heart attack

Frequently nothing much happens before a heart attack. The first signs of arterial disease having reached an advanced stage are, if you are lucky, severe chest pains, particularly during or soon after exercise or when under stress. This pain, which may also be felt down the left arm and up to the chin, is known as *angina pectoris* or more simply 'angina'. It is the pain of a heart in distress and it is serious because it is a very definite warning sign that a heart attack is a possibility and it is time to act.

The heart attack itself – what doctors call a *coronary thrombosis* or *acute myocardial infarction* – is the inevitable result of blocked arteries. The heart is intimately linked to both the brain and lungs and abnormalities in both can also cause it to seize up. Rare though this is, heart attacks nevertheless hit more than 600 people every day in Britain. A heart attack is not necessarily fatal but it is often disabling and full recovery is frequently difficult and uncertain, as much because of the psychological effects it has as any physical damage. By the time this stage is reached it is very often too late to do anything.

What makes heart disease so particularly difficult and distressing for most people is the notion that it is possible to feel perfectly well one minute and be dead the next. You jump from stage one to stage three, in other words, without any warning. The famous American keep-fit fanatic Jim Fix, author of the best-selling *Complete Book of Running*, dropped dead at 52 – while jogging – apparently with no idea he was in danger. All the signs commonly believed to give an indication of potential disaster weren't there.

There is, in fact, only a degree of truth in the idea of heart disease as a 'silent killer'. The warnings are usually there if you care to read them. The trouble is that most people, particularly men it has to be said (see also chapter 4), are highly skilful at pretending nothing is wrong. That is why it was said earlier you are lucky if you get 'stage 2' warning signs. They at least tell you that you are hitting your limits and so give you a chance to turn the tide in your favour before it's too late.

Other problems

Two further related problems can arise at the heart attack stage: the rhythm of the heart can be upset – called *arrhythmia* – and this is in fact a common cause of death in the early stages of a heart attack, and dangerous blood clots can form.

A blood clot, or *thrombus*, is a piece of thickened or congealed blood which is a major cause of sudden blockage leading to a heart attack. If a blood clot, which can form in thick sluggish blood at any time, reaches the brain and blocks any of the arteries supplying it with blood the result can be a **stroke**. The proper medical name for a stroke is a *cerebral thrombosis* or *cerebral infarction*. What happens is the part of the brain deprived of blood dies and so that part of the mind 'shuts down', resulting sometimes in death but more frequently in a form of paralysis and disability.

An alternative cause of stroke is the rupturing of the delicate arteries in the brain so that they bleed straight into the brain tissue. This is known as a *cerebral haemorrhage* and has much the same effect as a thrombosis.

A stroke is not, of course, a heart attack although the cause is the same. With a stroke you are aware something is wrong. It is perfectly possible to have a heart attack, however, without fully realizing it. In mild form there is no collapse and no pain worse than something you might take for indigestion. It is on record that some of the worst people for making this basic, and serious, mistake are doctors! The important thing is to recognize the few symptoms there may be for what they are and not just dismiss them. Arteries can be as much as 90 per cent blocked before symptoms of heart disease become obvious.

Why does heart disease develop?

We know that for the body to be perfectly healthy, for it to function at maximum efficiency, it is necessary above all for the blood to be 'just right', as Goldilocks would have said. That means it should have the right ingredients and consistency and move round the body at the right speed and pressure. We also know that we must have strong and supple blood vessels and a strong heart muscle. We are made to have all these things, and indeed most of us are born with them. So what goes wrong?

What goes wrong, as survey after survey has now shown conclusively, is that we lead unhappy and unhealthy lives. We eat too much, we eat the wrong things, we drink too much, we sit around too much, we don't exercise enough, we get angry, we smoke too much, we live in unhealthy surroundings, we are over-worked and underpaid and we get depressed! All these things not only place a strain on our heart and blood vessels but also release hostile chemicals into our bloodstream. Over a period of time – and obviously it varies from person to person (but the risk is highest in those with a family history of heart disease) – these chemicals damage the vessels so badly that they finally choke up and 'kill' the heart muscle.

Some of these factors are our own fault and others not at all of our own making, some we can do something about and others we can't, many are physical but many, importantly, are not: they are psychological – that is, they deal with our mental and emotional state. Most doctors know a lot about the physical factors but as many don't recognize, still less accept, the psychological ones. We'll come to those later. But first let's look at the factors everyone accepts.

Common signs of heart and blood vessel disease

The following are some of the most generally-recognized signs of heart and blood vessel disease but it is important to emphasize that having these symptoms is no more a guarantee you have heart disease than lack of them says you haven't. You can have heart disease without any obvious symptoms at all:

- angina (chest pain)
- leg cramps (known medically as 'intermittent claudication')
- poor circulation in legs ('peripheral ischaemia'), leg ulcers
- dizziness
- weakness
- breathlessness
- mental feebleness (for example, poor memory, mental confusion)
- weak pulse (or 'wide' pulse pressure)
- increasing clumsiness, lack of coordination, dexterity or agility
- ear-lobe crease.

The ear-lobe crease test

A diagonal crease in the ear-lobe *(see figure 2)*, first noticed in 1973 and now with some 30 medical studies in support, is one of the best indications yet discovered of heart disease. According to *The Encyclopaedia of Natural Medicine* it is 'a better predictor of heart disease than any other known risk factor...while [it] does not prove heart disease, it strongly suggests it'. The ear-lobe is particularly well supplied with blood and a drop in blood flow due to atherosclerosis leads to a collapse of blood vessels. This shows up as a well-defined crease which can be clearly seen as well as felt. The crease can be seen at any age but becomes more noticeable as you grow older (it seems to be less common after the age of 80). It is less reliable as an indicator among Asian or Oriental people or native Americans.

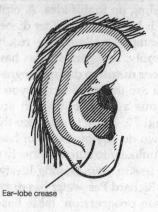

Ear-lobe crease

Figure 2 The ear-lobe crease

Who is most at risk, and when?

As we have already seen in the example of Jim Fix, a particularly unpleasant aspect of heart disease is that it can strike at anyone at any time, sometimes without much warning. But are some people more susceptible than others? The answer is yes. Researchers worldwide have now drawn up a pretty accurate profile of who is most at risk and when.

- Inherited characteristics and weaknesses, such as a family history of heart and blood disorders, are very important so-called 'risk factors'.
- People born with a family tendency towards high levels of blood fats – what doctors call *familial hyperlipidaemia* and *hypercholesterolaemia* – and high blood sugar (*diabetes*) are also considered particularly at risk. (Although most doctors believe that the defect is genetic – that is, it is 'programmed' into you and once you've got it you are stuck with it – there is some

challenge building up to this idea. A joint UK-Russian research team is looking at whether diabetes and heart disease, for example, really are the result of inherited genetics or simply, as recent studies have suggested, the result of poor nutrition during pregnancy.)

- The older you are the more at risk you become. The most dangerous age for both men and women is between 45 and 70. There is evidence that after 70, if you have shown no obvious signs of heart disease by then, you are unlikely to suffer seriously from it if you keep more or less to your existing lifestyle. American researcher Dr Richard Passwater has drawn up the following 'disease progression' table based on his 35 years observation:

Age range	Arterial deterioration
0-20	Fatty streaks develop
20-30	Fibrous plaque develops
25-40 plus	Calcification sets in
50 plus	Heart problems start

However, family tendency is a major determining factor here. The chances of developing heart disease in your twenties, or even teens, are high if both parents have the 'high fat' genes. If only one parent has the genes heart disease is still a strong possibility but a little later, in your forties and fifties.

- Men are far more prone to heart disease than women, but heart disease is increasing among women faster than among men and by the time a woman is past 65 or so she is even more likely to suffer from it than men. (Recently researchers have suggested the regular loss of iron through menstruation as a reason for the lower rate among premenopausal women but this remains unproven and it is more likely to do with the female hormone oestrogen.)

- Those in what experts like to call the 'lower socio-economic groups' – basically manual workers – suffer more heart disease than those in better-off groups.
- People of Asian origin are far more likely to be sufferers than other ethnic groups (although Afro-Caribbean people, particularly women, suffer more strokes than other groups).
- Scots and Northern Irish have the highest rate of heart disease in the world (see chapter 5).
- Those in demanding, boring, repetitive jobs have a greater chance of getting heart disease than those in less demanding, interesting and varied jobs (see chapter 4).
- People who don't exercise are at much greater risk than those who do, as are people who eats lots of sugar and fatty foods (see chapter 5).
- Meat-eaters are at three times the risk of non meat-eaters.
- Smokers are at higher risk than non-smokers.

All the above are what are called 'pre-disposing factors'. Each one you can tick off as applying to you multiplies your chances of getting heart disease considerably. In other words, your chances of getting heart disease over 50 are far higher if you are a meat-eating Asian male smoker with a family history of heart disease working in Scotland as a punch-card operator than a white female non-smoking bank clerk in London who loves fish. But it does not guarantee you will get heart disease any more than the bank clerk is guaranteed immunity. Other factors also play a major part, such as stress and high blood pressure.

But to understand more about this it is important first to know a bit more about how the heart and arteries work.

CHAPTER 2

All about your heart and arteries

How they work and why they're important

As explained in the last chapter we get heart disease basically because:

- Our blood is not 'clean' and fluid enough.
- Our arteries are not clear enough.
- Our heart is not pumping properly.
- Our arteries are narrowed by high levels of tension.

The important point about this is that heart, arteries and blood are all intimately linked. Together they make up what is known as the 'circulatory system'. This is the system which circulates blood around your body and it is a system at once both awe-inspiringly simple and vitally important.

First discovered in the 17th-century by the English physician William Harvey, the circulatory system can be compared to an intricate network of irrigation channels and canals watering an otherwise lifeless desert (*see figure 3*). The desert needs the water to stay green, fertile and healthy. The water is pushed rapidly around the system by a single highly efficient pump but any silting-up will result not only in the land becoming dry and eventually useless but will also damage the pump. So it is with the human body.

Blood vessels are like irrigation channels. Any interruption to the flow of blood means vital life-giving

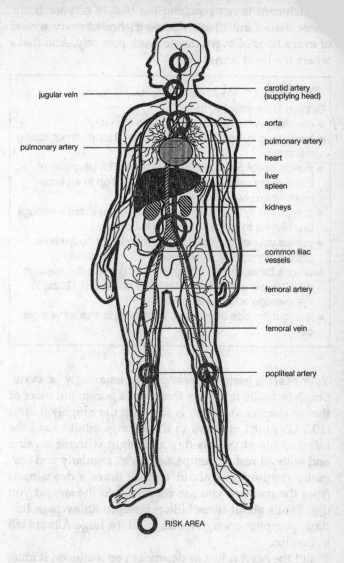

Figure 3 The circulatory system showing main 'risk areas'

t is not reaching the tissues of your body.
s must have that nourishment every second
r of every day to work properly. And that's
art comes in.

Heart facts

Did you know your heart:

- develops in the embryo around the 27th day
- beats roughly 100,000 times a day or 3 billion times during a lifetime
- pumps about 5 litres (9 imperial pints/10.5 US pints) of blood every minute when you rest – but up to six times more when you exercise
- pumps nearly 23,000 litres (5,000 gallons) a day – enough in a lifetime to fill the Albert Hall in London
- pumps your entire blood supply round your body about once every minute, but quicker if you rush about
- weighs between 230-280 grams (8-10ozs) in the average adult female and between 280-340 grams (10-12ozs) in the average adult male
- is about the size of your fist, increasing in size as you get older.

Your heart is basically a simple but amazingly powerful pump (actually it is more than 'just a pump' but more of that in chapter 4). Its job is to pump the roughly 5 litres (10.5 US pints) of blood in the average adult round the miles of blood vessels day and night without ceasing and without rest. It pumps, or 'beats', regularly and normally rhythmically about 100,000 times a day almost from the moment you are conceived to the second you die. That's about three billion times in an average lifetime, pumping enough blood to fill the huge Albert Hall in London!

But the heart is just as dependent on the blood it must pump round your body as the rest of you. It is basically a muscle and like any other muscle it must have blood to make it work and keep it healthy. If it gets starved of blood because of the silting up of blood vessels it starts to get 'rusty' and 'creaky' like some worn-out old engine with no oil. It will not pump so efficiently, and the silting up will get worse. So begins the vicious cycle of degeneration and decay that leads to what doctors call variously cardiovascular disease (CVD), coronary artery disease (CAD), coronary heart disease (CHD) and ischaemic heart disease (IHD) and what we are calling simply 'heart disease'.

But establishing that, like the twins Tweedledum and Tweedledee, the heart and the body's blood vessels are an inter-dependent and inseparable double-act misses out the single most important item in the whole process: blood itself. Just as the purpose of a pump and channels is to supply water to a dry landscape, and without the water the whole exercise becomes rather pointless, so blood is central to the purpose of the heart and blood vessels.

Blood has many vital functions, chief of which is to supply oxygen to every tissue in the body. Oxygen is essential to every one of the bodily processes which keep us alive; without it there is no life. It is the job of the heart and blood vessels to make sure blood reaches every part of the body and keep it on the move, fast. To follow how this happens it is worth understanding a little more about how blood is pumped round the body

How the heart works

As figure 4 shows, the heart is a two-sided pump, the left side pumping blood round the body and the right side pumping blood to the lungs. Blood leaving the heart passes out through vessels known as arteries (and eventually arterioles and capillaries) and returning to the

heart it travels through veins (and venules). Inside the
heart itself there are four chambers or 'reservoirs', two
on the right side and two on the left. Special one-way
valves between each of the chambers make sure the
blood flows in the same direction from one to the other.
Blood returning to the heart from the body enters the
heart through the right chamber (or 'atrium') and passes

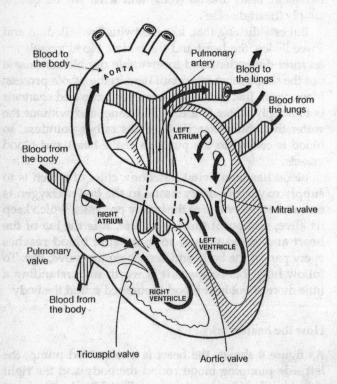

Figure 4 How the heart works
By courtesy of the British Heart Foundation

down into the chamber immediately below ɪ 'ventricle').

It is then pumped through the lungs (**out** through the pulmonary artery and **in** through the pulmonary veins) where it picks up the oxygen it circulates throughout the body from millions of tiny little blood-surrounded air sacs known as 'alveoli'. Blood from the lungs enters the heart through the left atrium, passes down into the left ventricle and from there it is pumped to all parts of the body. Figure 4 shows the cycle of events.

The importance of arteries

In a choice of which vessels are the most important arteries win out over veins every time. Arteries contain 'energy-rich' blood full of oxygen (from the lungs) leaving the heart to 'feed' every cell in your body while veins are only returning 'used' blood, empty of oxygen, to the heart (and the lungs) for 'recharging'. Arterial blood, full of oxygen, is bright red while blood in the veins, empty of oxygen, is dark red, almost brown.

The walls of both arteries and veins are made up of an inner lining, a layer of smooth elastic muscle-fibre and an outer coating. But because they have to take the full pressure of the heart pumping out, arteries have a much thicker layer of muscle and are therefore much thicker and stronger than veins. They are linked, as are all blood vessels – and indeed the heart itself – by an intricate network of nerves direct to the brain. This is important, as we'll see in chapter 4.

Most important of all, however, is the fact that it is the arteries that supply the heart muscle itself – the dynamic pump – with the oxygen it needs to work. This job is done by three main arteries on either side of the heart. As they appear to circle the heart they have been compared to a crown – hence the term 'coronary' (from the

for crown). It is when any of these arteries
red up' that a heart attack starts to become
becomes inevitable when they block up.

Did you know
● There are about 60,000 miles of blood vessels in your
  body, longer than all the roads of Scotland and Wales
  together.
● Blood travels at about 200mph (320kph) through the vessels of a healthy adult at rest but at more than 1,000mph
  (1,600kph) if taking vigorous exercise.
● The combined surface area of the several billion smallest
  blood vessels is the size of a soccer pitch.
● Your body produces some 100 billion red blood cells every
  day.
● Your body's total blood supply (5 litres or 10.5 US pints) is
  replaced roughly every four months.
● Blood 'soaks up' oxygen and 'dumps' cardon dioxide
  through the mass of tiny blood vessels (capillaries) sur-
  rounding each of the 300 million alveoli (air sacs) in the
  lungs.

The 'down' side to arteries is that they are subject to
much more strain from having to cope with the
continual pressure of blood being pumped through
them. (A severed artery is also extremely dangerous for
the same reason.) But it is this continual strain which
seems to be one of the main reasons arteries are more
liable to disease than veins. Veins remain relatively free
of disease throughout your life. Even though they
become less 'elastic' with age like arteries and the rest of
the body they do not get clogged up like arteries.
Surgeons who have used healthy veins to replace diseased arteries have found that after a time grafted veins
become just as clogged up and diseased as the replaced
arteries.

For the reason for this we need to look more closely at the nature of blood itself.

The importance of blood

To function at its best and keep you healthy the heart needs good clean blood. But the heart does not clean blood any more than it makes it. Blood, perhaps surprisingly, is made mainly by your bones – or more exactly by the marrow inside bones (and also by the lymph nodes and spleen: *see box on page 26*). The cleaning of blood takes place in the kidneys and spleen. Another vital organ is the liver which supplies the blood with many of its essential chemicals and acts as a kind of 'switching station'. Around 30 per cent of the blood in your body is in the liver at any given moment.

As we have already seen, the heart relies on a good clean supply of blood it can pump endlessly and regularly through itself to every part of your body through the blood vessels. Any sort of interruption or blockage in the tubing results in less effective circulation, and the poorer the circulation the greater the decline in energy, well-being and general health. But ageing is not the only reason why your blood vessels, in particular your arteries, get furred up. The nature of blood itself is the main cause.

What is blood?

Blood is an extraordinary substance. It is made up of a combination of fluids that together carry all the complex and subtle chemicals your body needs to function. There are about five litres (9 imperial pints, 10.5 US pints) in the average adult, consisting of roughly two-fifths red blood cells (*erythrocytes*) and three-fifths plasma, a semi-clear solution of proteins and mineral salts. There is also a small amount of white blood cells *(leukocytes)* and platelets. To 'work' properly blood must be of the right consistency and be constantly on the move. It quickly congeals or 'hardens' if left to stand.

Where blood is made

Blood is made mainly in bone marrow, particularly the marrow of long bones and the skull, backbone, ribs and breastbone, and also in the lymph nodes and the spleen.

Bone marrow produces red blood cells (which make up about two-fifths of all our blood supply and are the most numerous type of blood cells) as well as some white blood cells, which protect the body against infection, and clotting agents called *platelets*.

The *lymph nodes* and the *spleen* produce the rest of the white cells and together are an important part of the body's defense (or immune) system. The spleen, especially, is an interestingly complex little organ whose job, as well as to make white blood cells, is also to filter blood and remove old or damaged red blood cells.

The most important function of blood is to carry oxygen from the lungs to every cell in the body and bring back carbon dioxide gas to be released into the lungs. Oxygen is the basic fuel of life and its function in the body is to produce energy by 'burning' sugar and fat. Similarly, carbon dioxide is the waste product of that process. But this is far from all.

Blood also carries with it all the many other chemicals the body needs – from vitamins and minerals, proteins, fats and sugars to the vital hormones that are the body's own 'chemical controllers', controlling the body's essential activities. Blood also performs other functions, such as helping control body temperature, distributing salts the body's cells need to work properly, fighting infection and building up immunity.

But as well as performing helpful and necessary functions blood is capable of causing damage, particularly to artery walls, by carrying with it other less beneficial ingredients. We'll take a closer look at this next.

CHAPTER 3

Physical causes and risk factors

All about blood pressure and cholesterol

When doctors talk of 'major risk factors' in heart disease they usually mean smoking, lack of exercise and two more very specific items they always place at the top of any list. They are:

- High blood pressure (known as 'hypertension'), and
- High blood cholesterol.

Both high blood pressure and high blood cholesterol are known as 'blood risk factors'. Everyone has heard of them. Cholesterol, in particular, has become one the 'buzz' words of everyday speech. But even though everyone may have heard of them very few know exactly what they are and why they are 'bad'. In fact the situation is nowhere near as clear as you might think, and certainly not as clear as you are led to believe.

High blood pressure

Most doctors believe having blood pressure that is too high is an undisputed risk. About one person in ten with high blood pressure is unaware of it and yet it is a prime cause of stroke. Many life insurance companies base life expectancy predictions on nothing else but blood pressure readings. In fact having blood pressure that is too low is as serious as too high. So what is it and why is there so much emphasis on the problems of high blood pressure?

Blood pressure is the force the heart exerts to pump the body's five litres of blood around its 60,000 miles of blood vessels. If the arteries are even slightly narrowed the heart is under terrific strain to keep that blood flowing. The clearer the arteries the easier the heart's job. High blood pressure is one sign of narrowing arteries (atherosclerosis) and a call for action. Blood pressure is therefore an indication of the health of the heart and arteries.

Taking blood pressure

Blood pressure is read using a stethoscope and a sphygmomanometer, an inflatable arm 'cuff' attached to a mercury pressure gauge like an upright thermometer. It is difficult but not impossible to do your own reading in the same way you can take your own pulse. By inflating the 'cuff' on your left upper arm you effectively start cutting off the blood supply to your lower arm and automatically make the blood vessels in the arm swell up. Placing the 'bell' end of the stethoscope on the prominent artery in the crook of your arm listen for your pulse. Now inflate the cuff until you can no longer hear the pulse. *Slowly* release the pressure in the cuff until you hear the pulse return. Note the reading at that point. That is your systolic (maximum) pressure. Continue releasing pressure until the pulse fades to nothing. Again note the reading at that point. That is the diastolic (minimum) pressure. *To get a worthwhile reading take it at least three times at different times of the day both when you are resting and after exercising. The average of the three readings is likely to be your actual blood pressure.*

Factors that are likely to lead to high blood pressure or to aggravate the situation are being overweight, drinking too much alcohol and smoking. Women on the contraceptive pill can also be subject to high blood pressure.

Generally the older you are the higher readings get, especially when you leave your twenties. But it is still possible to have high blood pressure without being in any of these categories.

Blood pressure is measured by takings readings of the maximum and minimum strain the heart is under in pumping blood round your body. Measurements relate to the pulse. What you are feeling when you feel your pulse is the heart pumping. The pulse is the beat of the heart: a slow pulse is a slow heart beat, a fast pulse a fast beat. One beat is one pump of the heart muscle. A blood pressure reading measures the force in a single beat. So the first reading is the measurement of the force (measured in millimetres of mercury: mm/Hg) the heart is exerting when it beats, pumping blood out of your heart into your arteries. This is the maximum reading and it is called the *systolic* pressure. The bottom reading is the pressure between beats, when the heart is 'resting'. This is the minimum reading and it is the *diastolic* pressure.

The first thing to know is that there is no such thing as an 'ideal pressure' even though some people claim that the ideal is a reading of 120/80. Blood pressure varies for each person and it also varies constantly throughout the day, depending on your emotional state. It goes up when you are excited, angry or afraid – part of the so-called 'fight or flight' response, dating back to our prehistoric ancestors – and drops when you are relaxed. It would need to be checked regularly over a period of time to establish whether you had either a consistently high or low level, and also against whether any past members of your family lived healthily on either high or low blood pressure. Some people survive naturally on levels higher than the 120/80 'standard' and others on levels lower. There is no agreement on the 'right' level no matter what you may be told. Any reading over

160/100 or under 100/60 is probably a danger signal – in fact high blood pressure does not technically become the medical condition 'hypertension' until the reading is 160/100 or more.

Too high a systolic reading (over 160) may mean the heart is exhausting itself; too low (under 100) may mean the heart is weakening. Too high a diastolic reading (over 100), on the other hand, means the heart is under too much constant pressure and isn't getting enough rest; too low (under 60) may mean, again, a failing heart. Many people, especially women, seem to have a consistently low blood pressure associated with tiredness but it is not necessarily a symptom of heart failure.

A guide to blood pressure and pulse readings		
	'Normal' range	High risk
Blood pressure	100/60-140/90	Under 100/60
		Over 160/100
Pulse (at rest)	60-80 beats a min	Under 50 beats a min
		Over 100 beats a min

High blood cholesterol

But if there is disagreement about blood pressure there is even more over cholesterol. Cholesterol is not the only 'problem' substance in blood any more than it is the only substance. It is not even unique to blood. Cholesterol is a natural component of animal oils and fats, nerves, bile and egg yolk as well as blood. In blood it is just one of many substances the blood, and body, needs. Indeed it is essential. So the first important fact we need to understand about cholesterol is that it is fundamentally 'good', not 'bad' at all. Despite this it now has the reputation of being something akin to the big bad wolf in the heart disease story. Why is this?

Cholesterol is just one of many types of blood fats called *lipids*. It comes from the liver, where it is made, and also from what we eat. Other important lipids are *triglycerides*, which are linked particularly to the amount of refined carbohydrates such as sugar and starch we eat. They are both contained in the blood plasma, and together they are part of the blood's 'energy-chain' which feeds the body's cells.

The important thing we need to know about cholesterol in the blood is that it travels as two forms of lipoproteins – *high density lipoproteins* (HDL) and *low density lipoproteins* (LDL). High density lipoproteins are 'good guys' but low density lipoproteins are 'bad'. LDL-cholesterol, as it is called, is dangerous because it reduces levels of beta carotene (vitamin A) and vitamin E in the body and turns 'rancid' (oxidizes). This causes damage to cells in the lining of the arteries – and so arterial disease sets in. HDL-cholesterol, on the other hand, has a cleansing effect on blood and arteries and helps return good cholesterol to the liver where it is properly and harmlessly re-processed and expelled as bile. So the more cholesterol carried by HDL and the less by LDL the better.

Unfortunately, somewhere between 70-80 per cent of all cholesterol in the blood is LDL-cholesterol. The following table shows the ideal range of all blood fat levels including cholesterol. These blood tests, which show the balance between HDL and LDL, are very much more useful than measuring total levels. Figures that show total cholesterol levels alone are frankly misleading. Also they fail to take into account not only that cholesterol levels naturally increase with age and stress but also that there is a variation depending on your sex.

Ideal blood fat levels

		Europe	USA
HDL Cholesterol	Men	Minimum 0.8-1.9	30-75
	Women	Minimum 0.9-2.2	35-85
(The higher the better: ideal levels over 20% of total)			
LDL Cholesterol		Maximum 4.9	160
(The lower the better)			
Total Cholesterol	Under 60	Maximum 6.0	200
	Over 60	Maximum 7.0	235
Triglycerides		Maximum 2.0	180

European measurements in mmol per litre; US in mg/100ml.

The cholesterol riddle

Whether cholesterol is good or bad for you is a question doctors and scientists have been arguing over since the last century and is still undecided. New studies are being produced all the time that switch the argument first one way and then the other. The latest study by a team at St Bartholomew's Hospital in London, published in January 1994, moved the argument against cholesterol testing. The team, headed by Professor Nicholas Wald, concluded that cholesterol was not as important as lifestyle in the prevention of heart disease. In fact the case against cholesterol has been crumbling for about 20 years – though you are not told this.

'The relevance of a low cholesterol level [in preventing heart disease] is still in doubt', said a US family medical encyclopaedia published in 1979. Ten years later prize-winning British researcher Dr Richard Totman was still remarking: 'There can be no doubt that recommendations about saturated fats and cholesterol in the diet, and about their effect on cholesterol in the blood and heart disease, have been far too eager. Too much has been said based on too premature an interpretation, and often a misinterpretation, of the facts. Proclaiming, declaiming and denouncing have for some reason, perhaps political, perhaps commercial, taken over from reasoned reporting and have led to a serious misleading of the public.'

Citing a total of 19 studies carried out over 31 years it said had failed to establish that lowering cholesterol levels prevents heart attacks, the campaigning UK magazine *What Doctors Don't Tell You* in 1993 concluded also: 'There's no real evidence that raised cholesterol levels actually cause heart attack.' According to Dr Dean Ornish, one of the world's leading heart specialists, when people with heart disease follow a low cholesterol diet (30 per cent 200 milligram cholesterol), as officially recommended by the American Heart Association, 'the majority get worse rather than better'.

So it is curious in the extreme not only that almost all official advice still cites high cholesterol in the blood as an undisputed risk factor in heart disease and supports the use of a whole range of cholesterol-lowering drugs and diets, but also that commercially-produced cholesterol testing kits have started flooding the market.

The truth is that the amount of cholesterol the body takes in from what we eat is small and the body seems to have a sort of take-it or leave-it attitude towards it. In 1991 Professor Matthew Muldoon of Pittsburgh University carried out a review of all the trials of cholesterol-lowering drugs (which interfere artificially with the liver) and found that far from doing good they actually seemed to be harmful. Among the most serious side-effects he showed they caused were severe depression, leading to personality changes, violent behaviour and suicide.

So if a majority of people who suffer heart attacks do not have greatly elevated cholesterol levels who or what is the real culprit? Growing numbers of specialists are now starting to confirm that the immediate cause of arterial disease – which lies behind heart disease – is most probably neither cholesterol nor fats in general but a very specific combination of 'free radicals' and a particular type of LDL (bad) cholesterol called *lipoprotein-a*.

Free radicals, lipoprotein-a and heart disease

Research has been going on among pioneer nutritionists since the early 1960s into the action in the human body of *free radicals*. Free radicals are unruly little particles that run riot in the body gobbling up everything in sight. British biochemist Professor David Blake has called free radicals 'the most powerful toxin (poison) in the body' and 'a powerful system of destruction'. It now seems there is a significant link between free radicals and lipoprotein-a.

The theory is a simple one: Ageing in the human body is exactly like iron going rusty or butter going rancid. It is a process known as 'oxidation'. Oxygen is essential for life but in the wrong conditions it has the opposite effect. Free radicals are single 'hungry' oxygen molecules that biochemists know as *hydroxils*. In the wrong conditions they cause oxidation by binding to healthy cells and effectively sending them out of control by damaging their nucleus. The cells may then run amok, which is what happens in cancer, or shut down. Free radicals particularly like fats, and their relevance to heart disease is that fats are an essential part of what makes cells flexible, including of course the cells of the blood, heart and arteries.

Lipoprotein-a is the product of cholesterol after it has been turned rancid (oxidized). The discovery of a Norwegian researcher, lipoprotein-a seems to act like some sort of outlaw gang leader, stimulating hordes of delinquent free radicals to pillage and vandalize the body. Free radicals are actually an essential part of the body's self-repair mechanism. Their job is to kill bacteria. But lipoprotein-a seems to have the power to turn them against the body instead and send them on the rampage. Recent German research has shown that arterial plaques are composed almost entirely of lipoprotein-a.

Lipoprotein-a is normally low in healthy blood but high levels of lipoprotein-a (and not necessarily high levels of cholesterol) are now believed to be a guarantee of arterial disease. According to pioneer American researcher Professor Linus Pauling, winner of two Nobel Prizes for his work in nutrition, more than 20 milligrams per litre of lipoprotein-a in the bloodstream is deadly. *Leading specialists are now saying that the really important blood test is therefore not cholesterol but lipoprotein-a.*

How blood 'nasties' damage the arteries

The walls of healthy arteries are smooth to allow blood to flow swiftly through. For lipoprotein-a – or any damaging element in the blood – to lodge itself and build up it has to have something to lodge onto. A key role here is the action of another little nasty called *homocystine*.

Homocystine is a spin-off from the essential amino acid *methionine*. Amino acids are part of the protein process of making cells in the body and methionine is critically involved in brain, liver, kidney and fat function. Homocystine is produced when methionine does not 'convert' properly (thought to be due to a vitamin B6, pyridoxine, deficiency). It then acts like a sort of chemical 'sandpaper', scratching and scouring the smooth walls of the blood vessels, but particularly the arteries. The cuts and grooves it makes attract every piece of undesirable debris in the blood, including nasties such as lipoprotein-a, and gives them a firm foothold – and so the atheromous buildup starts. (For more on amino acids and the causes and cures of homocystine built-up see chapter 9.)

Testing for blood 'nasties'

Special blood tests can establish the levels of unwelcome ingredients such as lipoprotein-a and homocystine. The British heart charity the Arterial Health Foundation (AHF), which supports gentle treatments for heart disease, advises asking your doctor for a *full blood profile* if you suspect you have heart disease. This gives not only your full blood count (red and white cell count) but also the complete biochemical profile of your blood, including the level of fats present and liver and kidney function. It should include not only an analysis of all the so-called 'risk factors' including cholesterol but show the precise individual readings for HDL and LDL cholesterol, triglycerides, lipoprotein-a, and homocystine. If your family doctor does not know what you are talking about (which is likely) remind him or her that professional analysis laboratories know about such tests and should be able to carry them out as a routine exercise if asked.

According to the charity any readings for lipoprotein-a above 2g per litre or for homocystine above 5mmol per litre – the ideal is zero in both cases – is a sign for immediate action to stop and reverse almost certain arterial damage. (Remember, you are entitled to see the results of your tests and to ask for a copy.) For more details contact the AHF *(see Appendix A)*.

The 'secret' of antioxidants

Talking to an international audience in London in November 1993 pioneer American researcher Dr Richard Passwater said he believed there is no mystique about why heart disease develops or how to prevent and cure it: 'What I can tell you about beating heart disease is exactly what my mom used to say, and it is as true today as it was then – eat well, eat a varied diet, eat in moderation, take plenty of exercise and take vitamins and minerals.'

To him heart (or rather arterial) disease is basically a disease not of ageing but of malnutrition. Dr Passwater, director of a nutrition research centre in Maryland, is one of a handful of pioneers, including former colleague Professor Pauling, who have maintained for more than 30 years that most doctor's increasing obsession with drugs and surgery to treat heart disease is both misguided and unnecessary. They have been the pioneers of research into 'antioxidants'.

If free radicals are the body's villains antioxidants are its heroes. Antioxidants are nutrients that round up free radicals and destroy them. Like rust-proofing on a car, they are 'conserving' nutrients. The mayfly lives for barely a day or two because it has virtually no antioxidants. Animals that live to a ripe old age have not only a low metabolism but also possess very good antioxidant protection. Antioxidants can be vitamins (like vitamin C), minerals (like zinc) or amino acids (like lysine). All can be taken as 'food supplements' in powder, liquid or pill form. They can also be injected.

But despite being well researched, with literally hundreds of trials showing enormous success in both protecting against and treating heart disease, the vast majority of doctors and scientists have refused to believe or accept until very recently that there was the slightest connection between what we eat (and don't eat) and disease. Until recently they had barely heard of either free radicals or antioxidants (some still haven't!). They were even less inclined to believe that taking supplements was good or even necessary. A favourite taunt, repeated still by arch opponents, was that all you got was 'expensive urine'.

They were equally sceptical about another central claim of those who now think free radicals are central to the heart disease story: that what causes free radicals to run riot in the body is almost everything around us from environmental pollution – too much heat, sun, radiation, smoke, the wrong food and drink, bad air and water – to the waste products of the body itself and our own stress processes.

Slowly but surely, however, the evidence is mounting and the tide of opinion turning. This book is yet more evidence of it. Dr Passwater told his London audience how 30 years ago when he spoke about his work at a meeting in Washington to America's top scientists and doctors, members of the National Academy of Sciences, four people turned up. In November 1993 he spoke again, this time to a packed conference. One of the incentives was probably his claim that he can save $8.7 billion a year in hospital bills by the treatment of heart disease with antioxidants. But in Britain the government is now spending millions of pounds researching the benefits of antioxidants led by Professor Anthony Diplock, head of a special free radical research group set up at Guy's Hospital in London.

Professor Diplock's public pronouncements have so far been cautious in favour of the benefits. Dr Passwater has no such reservations. He told his London conference that antioxidants have the potential to 'aggressively inhibit the atheroma process', and predicted 'the next decade will significantly lower the incidence of cardio-vascular disease'. Among the most important antioxidants he identified was vitamin E – and its lack in the body as 'the single most important risk factor' in heart disease. In 10 years time low vitamin E may well be listed as a major medical risk factor. At the moment, however, that list is rather different.

Correcting blood levels naturally

The Arterial Health Foundation recommends the following action to help correct the levels of your blood 'risk factors' (see also chapter 9):

Cholesterol Stop eating all refined foods, hydrogenated fats (like margarine) and fried foods. Reduce your alcohol consumption to a minimum, increase the amount of (clean) water you drink and take more exercise. There are also a number of supplements you can take, in particular vitamin C and garlic, but consult a good natural health practitioner for the best advice on this.

Homocystine Supplement your diet with folate, vitamins B12 and B6 (pyridoxine), and the digestive enzyme betaine built into a single complex dose especially formulated for arterial disease. See a specialist practitioner about this such as a good naturopath.

Lipoprotein-a Take a good antioxidant formula supplement containing vitamins A, C, E, beta carotene and the minerals manganese, zinc, copper, selenium and molybdenum. Of these, vitamins C and E are the most valuable. Take 3-6 grams of vitamin C a day (250mg chewable tablets eaten regularly throughout the day are ideal) and at least 400iu vitamin E.

Other tests you can ask for are:

Ferritin This test measures the level of iron in your blood. Too high a reading (over 250ng/ml for men, 80ng/ml for women), suggesting you are taking in too much iron, is a danger signal because iron is a heavy metal and too much is as bad for you – if not worse – as too little. Iron is as toxic in excess as lead, mercury and cadmium. Eat more garlic, onions, zinc, copper and fibre.

Fibrinogen This is the level of fibrous material responsible for artery clotting. Again, if the reading is too high (over 4g/l) try adding foods high in omega-3 fatty acids (found in fish like tuna, sardines, herring and in cold pressed virgin olive oil) and eat less saturated fat. Remember that in this respect butter is better than margarine as long as it is still within the limits of your total saturated fat intake. An alternative is to take a regular EPA fish oil supplement (there are many excellent ones on the market).

Red cell magnesium Unlike the previous readings the higher the next two the better. If red cell magnesium is low – the ideal is to aim for a reading over 2.7 – increase your consumption of brown rice and vegetables, especially of green leaf varieties. Check your stress response with biofeedback and improve your colon health over a period since it is likely to be functioning poorly. If you cannot open your bowels normally at least once a day you could benefit from having colonic irrigation (washing of the colon) from a qualified practitioner (see chapter 9). Follow this with supplementation with acidophilus to increase the amount of healthy bacteria in the gut (take between meals 1-5 times a day, as directed by a health practitioner).

Serum E If the reading for serum E, the amount of vitamin E in your blood, is low – ideally it should be over 1.6mg% – start taking between 800-1000iu a day, together with omega-3 and omega-6 fatty acid (EPA and GLA) capsules. Absorption in the gut is helped by a tablespoon of flaxseed (linseed) oil taken either first thing in the morning or last thing at night or as a salad dressing *(NB Always buy flaxseed oil in darkened bottles. Once opened put in 1200iu of vitamin E to stop it going rancid and place it in the darkest part of the fridge)*. Again, as with red cell magnesium, check for stress response with biofeedback (find a health practitioner with the equipment). Stress produces fatty acids which destroy natural body oils.

(Abridged from AHF newsletter No5, 1993, with permission)

CHAPTER 4

Psychological causes and risk factors

How what you think and feel affects your heart

So far we have looked almost entirely at the physical picture. But there is another side to the story that is at least as important and, in the view of some experts, may even be more so: how what we think and feel affects our heart and arteries.

There is a reluctance to admit to the importance of 'feelings' and 'thoughts' in western society with its emphasis on mechanics and materials but it is still surprising how slow medicine generally has been to recognize its significance (as in the case of those doctors who say some illness is 'all in the mind' and give you a pill to send you away). For medically speaking there is nothing new about it. Modern heart research virtually started with the work of Dr Thomas Lewis, a London clinician who during the first world war investigated the phenomenon of 'soldier's heart'. He found that soldiers on the western front accused of malingering because they were collapsing for no apparent reason were simply reacting to the horrors of trench warfare. Their hearts couldn't take the emotional and mental strain of it all. Doctors called it 'neurosis'.

Unfortunately this direct link between our mental and emotional state – what we can call our psychological state – and our physical state seems to have become largely forgotten or buried in the rapid development this century of technological medicine – at least until recently. The evidence is now pretty conclusive: what you think and feel can, and does, affect your body, your blood, your skin, your tissues, your cells, your blood vessels, your brain, your lungs and all your other organs – including your heart. The evidence provides us with one of the most important insights into the causes of heart disease.

The 'feeling' heart

Describing the heart as a pump is convenient because it explains what the heart does fairly accurately. But it does not explain what the heart *is*. The heart is in fact much more than 'just a pump'. It is a muscle and because it is a muscle it is, like all muscles, linked to the brain by nerves – as is the entire circulatory system, veins, arteries and all. It is fairly obvious, therefore, that like any other part of the body surrounded and interwoven with nerves the heart and its blood vessels 'feel' in the same way your skin 'feels'. But this is not all. Because they are directly and powerfully linked to your brain and its senses they respond to pleasure, pain, anger, joy, despair, anxiety, disappointment and all the other emotions the human being is capable of feeling. They expand when you are relaxed and happy and contract when you are frightened and angry.

It is this important fact that has led to the description of the heart as a 'feeling organ'. This feeling aspect is expressed in a host of well-known sayings linking the heart with our emotions: 'My heart shrank with fear', 'burst with joy', 'broke into a thousand pieces' and so on. This accurately describes what happens to the heart muscle and the muscles encasing the blood vessels, and especially the arteries, when you experience almost any sort of emotion.

The famous American cardiologist (heart specialist) Dr Dean Ornish has pointed out that when we get angry, for example, our heart rate and blood pressure go up, our arteries may constrict and our blood may thicken and clot. It is small wonder, therefore, that anger is a well-known cause of heart attack.

Another American, the psychologist Alexander Lowen, believes the 'feeling' heart is one of the three 'vital and sentient' organs of the body: the others being the brain (the body's 'thinking' organ) and the genitals (its sexual organs). Moreover he has claimed the heart is the 'channel of communication' between the three, communicating through the throat and mouth, the arms and hands, and finally the genitals. All three sets of channels are capable of affecting the heart for better or worse via the nerves and brain.

He, like modern pioneer the British cardiologist Dr Peter Nixon, believes a heart can actually 'break' – not literally into separate pieces but it can become 'disconnected' and isolated from the rest of the body. As Lowen, founder of the therapeutic system Bioenergetics, poetically puts it: 'The feeling of love no longer flows freely from the heart to the world.'

The type A personality and the 'hostility factor'

Though it was probably obvious to most people all along it was not really until the 1960s that the first real scientific evidence for the mind-body connection started to appear. And interestingly the first pioneers were two cardiologists. Dr Meyer Friedman and Dr Ray Rosenman from San Francisco identified a group of characteristics they claimed were present in most of their heart patients: a tendency to be in a constant hurry, intense competitiveness and repressed anger – what the two doctors called 'free-floating hostility'. They coined the term

'Type A Personality' to define this type of person.

Later work, in the 1970s and 1980s, modified this rather simple model but did not undo it. The most striking thing Friedman and Rosenman discovered, in a study of 3,000 middle-aged men over nearly nine years, was that type A men are twice as likely to develop heart disease as the non-type As. More than this, not only did their study confirm the 'smoking, drinking, fat-eating' physical risk factors for heart disease found in an earlier major study in Massachusetts (the famous Framingham Study), but *they also found that type A men were more likely to get heart disease even if they fell into none of the physical risk factors.*

In 1980 a team of scientists at Duke University, North Carolina, published research that showed that of the three personality traits identified by Friedman and Rosenman it was only one – 'free-floating hostility' – which was really to blame for heart disease. It was a logical finding: hurrying and being competitive can be positive attributes and therefore beneficial whereas hostility is almost totally negative. In their test, using an extensive questionnaire known in academic circles as the Minnesota Multiphasic Personality Inventory (MMPI), the Duke team found that 70 per cent of patients who had high 'hostility' scores had severe artery blockages whereas half those with low scores had no blockages at all.

Other studies found much the same, sometimes dramatically so. Another Duke University researcher, psychologist Dr John Barefoot, looked at North Carolina doctors and lawyers 25 years after they had filled in the MMPI questionnaire as students and found that 'high hostility' doctors had four to five times more heart disease than low scores. In fact, he found that 14 per cent of the doctors and 20 per cent of the lawyers who had scored 'high hostility' when they were 25 were dead by the age of 50. Among the low-scoring students, by contrast, only two percent of doctors and four per cent of lawyers had died by the same age.

Hostility and sudden death

A further study of the lawyers defined the reasons rather more specifically than just general hostility. It found that the group had 'a cynical mistrust of people in general, the frequent experience of anger, and the overt expression of aggressive behavior'. In other words cynicism, aggression and having a 'short-fuse' were identified as risk factors. Other characteristics the researchers thought might be contributory factors in heart disease such as being nervous, paranoid and shy did *not* lead to a higher death rate.

Stanford University psychiatrist Dr Gail Ironson found in another study that asking heart patients to call to mind something in the past that had made them angry caused their heart blood supply to drop and their hearts to pump less well – a reduction that could lead to a sudden heart attack. Harvard Medical School psychologist Dr Richard Verrier has also shown that acute stress can cause dangerous abnormalities in the rhythm of the heart. Dr Nixon believes a sense of defeat is also a key factor in sudden heart attack. 'Coronary catastrophe', he says, is 'the union of rage with despair'. In other words, the body's normal 'fight or flight' responses – part of what biologists call the sympathetic and parasympathetic nervous systems – clash and crash.

Dr Redford Williams, director of the Behavioral Medicine Research Center at Duke University and head of its division of behavioral medicine, believes bottled-up anger, long suspected as a cause of illness, 'may increase the levels of stress hormones circulating in the blood which can have a number of long-term effects on the cardiovascular system'.

According to Dr Williams there are now 'many reports in the medical literature of sudden death precipitated by intense emotional stress'. One of the first such records, he believes, may have been the deaths of Ananias and his wife Sapphira about 2,000 years ago as described in the New Testament. Their instant deaths on being confronted with the accusation of cheating over money would be described today as 'sudden cardiac death bought on by acute, massive stress'. In fact, he says, it was probably due to 'an immense surge of the stress hormone adrenalin'.

Key psychological risk factors

- aggression
- anger
- anxiety
- cynicism
- high job stress
- loneliness/low social support
- defeat
- despair

The action of stress hormones

The release of too many stress hormones like *adrenalin* and *cortisol* can work the heart muscle so hard it basically collapses with exhaustion. In the words of Dr Williams, 'its cells curdle'. He is now convinced it is the action of stress hormones which is the key to the mind-body link between what we feel and heart disease.

American psychologist Dr Edward Suarez has found that men and women with high hostility scores show much larger increases in blood pressure and stress hormones when harassed than those with low hostility ratings. Higher than average amounts of adrenalin have also been found in the daytime urine of high hostility people (but not at night, suggesting it is a response to the stresses of the day). Adrenalin seems to

Test your hostility level

Tick the boxes if your answer is yes to any of the questions below. If it is no leave it as it is. Answer quickly and be honest.

- Do you count the number of items in people's baskets ahead of you in the supermarket 'express' checkout line to see they are within the limit? ☑
- Do you wonder who is holding up the lift (elevator) if it doesn't arrive as quickly as you think it should? ☑
- Do you frequently check up on other people when you've given them a job to make sure they're doing it properly? ☐
- Do you get easily and quickly worked up if you are held up in traffic or out shopping? ☑
- Do you feel like lashing out when even little things go wrong? ☐
- Do you quickly feel annoyed when someone criticizes you? ☐
- Do you bang the door or wall if you are kept waiting too long for a lift (elevator)? ☐
- Do you look for an opportunity to 'pay someone back' or 'get even' if they do something to you you don't like? ☐
- Do you get heated and talk or even mutter at the TV when there's something on you don't approve of or agree with? ☑

If your have ticked 'yes' to more than one question in each of the three groups (testing your cynicism, anger and aggression) or more than four questions overall you probably have a high hostility level and should take action to bring it down (see chapters 5 and 8). This is not a scientific test but gives you some idea of where you stand.

Based on a similar test in 'Mind-Body Medicine' (Consumer Reports Books, New York, 1993).

be particularly important.

'Adrenalin is known to raise blood pressure, make the blood clot more rapidly, and accelerate a host of other physiological processes that are likely to speed the growth of atherosclerotic plaques, including triggering the movement of fat from the body's fat stores into the bloodstream,' claims Dr Williams. Specifically, he believes the frequent surges of adrenalin experienced by high hostility people account for their generally higher than average cholesterol levels – because cholesterol also shoots up when we are under stress.

The part played by the brain

American researchers have found that as well as being aggressive and angry high hostility people tend to smoke more, eat more, drink more alcohol, be more overweight, have higher levels of 'bad' cholesterol (the LDL cholesterol) and lower of the 'good' (HDL). They also have low levels of *serotonin*.

Serotonin is one of the most important chemicals in the brain. It is a *neurotransmitter* and neurotransmitters are chemical 'messengers' that carry chemical 'messages' from one nerve to another. Serotonin is known to be crucially involved in the control of behaviour, but low serotonin is now thought to be the direct result of low levels of cholesterol – since cholesterol is an essential part of all cells in the body including the brain. But as we saw in the last chapter cholesterol *as* lipoprotein-a is involved in the formation of arterial plaques (atheromas) by the action of free radicals.

So now we have a situation in which too little cholesterol is as likely to lead to the physical damage of the heart and arteries as too much by setting up a sort of vicious cycle of physical and psychological cause-and-effect in which hostility and aggression – 'bad stress' – is central. In other words, psychological stress becomes not just a trigger but the main trigger of the many physical causes, including the production of lipoprotein-a, that can lead directly to heart disease.

Causes of stress

Convinced that 'stress seems to play a subtle long-term role in the development of coronary heart disease overall', Dr Williams' centre at Duke University is now one of some 10 research centres across America investigating the role of psychological and social issues in heart disease. Their work so far has confirmed those 'psychosocial risk factors' that can lead to heart disease and contribute to making it worse once it is there. As well as a hostile personality, they include job strain and lack of social support:

- *Job strain* American and Swedish researchers have shown that people in jobs that force them to work and concentrate hard with little control over what they are doing or how they do it have a much greater chance of developing heart disease and are more likely to die earlier because of it. Higher than normal blood pressure seems to be the main reason (*see figure 5*).
- *Social support* Much the same evidence has been found with people who lack a strong network of family and friends to support them. Several studies over many years have found more heart disease, and more deaths from heart disease, among the lonely than among those with good social support.

In one study 1,350 people with heart disease were followed over five years – and regardless of their degree of disease or physical risk factors *three times* more of those without someone to talk to, confide in and hug died compared with those with close support. Another study by three New York hospitals found that those patients living alone were twice as likely to have another attack within six months as those living with a partner or companion. Significantly, US psychologist Dr Andrew Baum has found that people living alone produce more adrenalin than those with close support.

By far the most dramatic study, however, is the now famous and continuing one being carried out by Dr Ornish at the University of California in San Francisco. Using people with severe heart disease divided randomly into two groups he has shown that those in the group following a programme with a purely low-fat diet, exercise, yoga and social support are not only better than the group having conventional heart treatment but their heart disease is actually reducing. Those in the group having the conventional treatment, on the other hand, have worse disease. (He also pointed out that people with heart disease who followed a specifically cholesterol-reducing diet, as recommended by the American Heart Association, get worse rather than better.)

Dr Ornish, whose research programme is the first to show that heart disease can be reversed simply by lifestyle modification without the use of drugs and surgery, is adamant that people who feel isolated have up to five times the death rate of those who feel supported. He has stated that in America he feels there is 'a real yearning for community' – and this may well be one of the most important reasons for the relatively low level of heart disease in southern European countries where community life is still strong compared with other parts of Europe and North America. Social support on its own, he believes, is among the very best forms of stress management because being part of a supportive group gives people 'a sense of meaning, empowerment and control over their lives' – which is what most people need, particularly men.

How stressful is your job?

The chart opposite, based on an actual survey of 4,500 American men and women, shows how likely you are to suffer from 'job stress' and therefore to be more at risk of developing heart disease. The horizontal line represents the demands put on you, from left to right, and the vertical line the degree of freedom you have to make your own decisions, with least freedom at the bottom and most at the top. For example, among the most stressful jobs are assembly-line worker, key-puncher and garment-stitcher and the least stressful architect and natural scientist.

What about women?

Research has shown that though men are twice as likely to die of heart disease, and six times more likely to die of a heart attack than women, women seem to be just as much at risk from psychological factors as men. The reason for their generally lower rate of heart disease seems to have a great deal to do with the 'female' hormone oestrogen. This protection disappears after the menopause – post-menopausal women over 75 actually suffer more heart disease than men and are more likely to die of it, particularly from stroke (more than twice as likely in fact) – but nevertheless the idea that women are somehow psychologically stronger than men is only partly born out by the evidence.

Depression, pessimism and 'domestic trauma', traditionally attributed more to women, have been shown to play little part in heart disease. Women may be naturally better at being on their own and 'coping' than men (despite their self-image, men seem less suited to being alone and may produce more stress hormones as a direct result: British research has shown that divorced men are twice as likely to die early as married men) but when

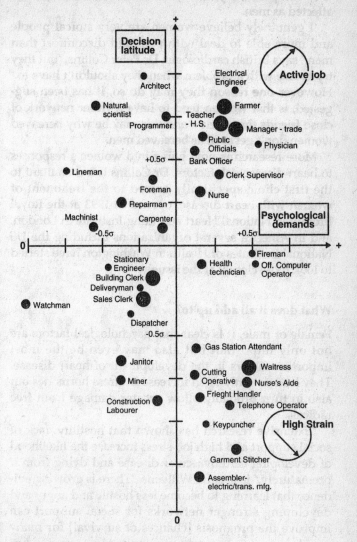

Figure 5 How stressful is your job?
By courtesy of Baywood Publishing Co.

they are positively lonely women seem to be just as affected as men.

'I genuinely believe women are very stoical people and more able to deal with pain and discomfort than men,' says British cardiologist Dr Peter Collins, 'but they try to live with a problem when they shouldn't have to.' However one reason they may do so, it has been suggested, is that women tend to have a wider network of close friends than men – and this may be why bereaved women don't get as ill as bereaved men.

More research is now going into women's responses to heart disease risk factors. Dr Collins is a consultant to the first clinic specifically geared to the treatment of women with heart disease, opened in 1993 at the Royal Brompton National Heart and Lung Institute in London, and in America several organizations including the US National Institutes of Health in Washington have started to look more closely at the issue.

What does it all add up to?

Female or male, it is clear that psychological factors are not only important but also may even be the most important factors in the development of heart disease. They lead not only to an increase in stress hormones but also in turn probably allow greater damage from free radicals.

'Extensive research has shown that hostility, lack of social support and high job stress increase the likelihood of developing cardiovascular disease and dying from it prematurely,' insists Dr Williams. 'There is growing evidence that learning to become less hostile and angry and developing stronger networks for social support can improve the prognosis [chances of survival] for many people.'

CHAPTER 5

How to help yourself

Rules and guidelines for preventing heart disease

The process of arterial deterioration leading to heart disease starts from birth (and even before it) and is generally regarded as an inevitable part of growing old. In fact there is nothing inevitable about it. Age clearly plays a part but the many assumptions made about the ageing process are now being questioned, especially in the light of what we know about the effects of increasing pollution as well as basic lifestyle on our health – and hearts.

The best and most natural way to beat heart disease is, of course, to avoid it in the first place. On this doctors and therapists on all sides, both conventional and unconventional, seem agreed. Prevention is better than cure, and nowhere is this more true than when applied to heart disease. Heart disease is not only one of the major causes of death and disability in the world it is also largely preventable. According to US cardiologist Dr Dean Ornish, one of the world's leading pioneers of gentle treatments for heart disease, as much as 95 per cent of heart disease is preventable.

This chapter is basically about helping yourself through prevention, but it is also about reversing heart disease. That is, *curing* it. The natural way with heart disease is essentially the way of prevention, and much the same principles apply in prevention as in the treatment of heart disease. Pioneers like Dr Ornish have shown that following most of the advice in this chapter can actually turn the clock back on heart disease. For just as we know that an artery has to be almost totally blocked before you feel any adverse effect Dr Ornish has pointed out that 'even a small change in a critically-blocked artery has a relatively big effect on blood flow to the heart'. So helping yourself to prevention is also helping yourself to curing heart disease if you already have it.

Helping yourself is actually easier said than done but at least there seems to be general agreement about what to do if not necessarily the ways or the order of doing it.

The Seven 'Deadly Sins'

- bottling-up feelings, particularly of aggression, and/or being under continual strain
- eating poor quality food (high-fat, refined, salty, sugary)
- eating little or no fresh fruit, vegetables or fish
- being overweight
- taking no exercise
- smoking
- drinking heavily

See tables on pages 60-72 for guidelines and targets.

The above list reflects the priorities outlined in this book. The order would not be agreed with by all doctors, and nor would the majority of doctors, few of whom are taught nutrition or psychology as part of their training, rate diet or stress as very significant. The latest evidence, however, is that nothing else – including smoking – is so significant *as a primary cause of heart disease.*

Britain, for example, and within Britain Scotland and Northern Ireland in particular, has some of the highest incidence of heart and arterial disease in the world. Compared with its European neighbour France, where smoking is popular, Britain has three times more deaths from heart disease for men aged 35-74 and nearly five times more deaths for women. World Health Organisation (WHO) statistics show clearly that Europe's other Mediterranean countries, Italy, Spain, Portugal and Greece, where smoking is also common, all have a far better record than not only Britain but also the northern European countries as a whole. Heart deaths in southern Europe are in fact on average *half* those of northern Europe.

Death rates in Europe from heart disease per 100,000 people for men and women aged between 35-74.

	Women	Men	Total
Southern Europe			
France	37	137	174
Greece	70	220	290
Italy	61	201	262
Portugal	60	162	222
Spain	37	168	205
Average	**53**	**178**	**231**
Northern Europe			
Belgium	87	257	344
Denmark	140	403	543
England & Wales	173	461	634
Germany	96	299	395
Ireland	193	543	736
Luxembourg	76	280	356
Netherlands	95	314	409
Northern Ireland	226	595	821
Scotland	173	605	778
Average	**140**	**417**	**557**
Overall average	**109**	**332**	**441**

Source: World Health Statistics Annuals 1989.

A string of surveys has now clearly highlighted that one of the major differences between the two regions, apart of course from sunshine, a more relaxed way of life and a strong sense of community, is diet. People in Mediterranean countries are not only avid smokers but also commonly eat large amounts of food known to promote a healthy cardiovascular system such as fish, fresh fruit and vegetables, olive oil, garlic and red wine. Long lunches are traditionally followed by a *siesta* (rest). The populations of Scotland and Northern Ireland, by contrast, eat the least amount of fruit and vegetables in the United Kingdom, the most sugar and often seem to live under the most unhealthy type of stress. An official 1992 study in Scotland found that 15 per cent of male manual workers never eat green vegetables and almost a quarter never eat fresh fruit. A similar story can be told elsewhere.

Why heart disease is a 'disease of civilization'

Barely 30 years ago the United States, now with a far better record than Britain, had death statistics similar to those in Scotland and Northern Ireland today. In 1968 some 800 people per 100,000 of the population of America died from heart disease. By 1986 that figure had dropped to 375, on a par with Germany now. The vast majority of the more than two million Americans who died every year of heart and arterial disease succumbed, according to US health authorities, through smoking and poor eating habits. Too much fat, sugar and refined foods were the main culprits. About a million Americans still die each year from heart disease but one difference between 1968 and 1986 was that the US government, spurred on by hard-hitting campaigners like Philip Sokoloff, founder of the National Heartsavers Association, introduced a major national prevention

drive aimed at the food industry to cut do
ated fats and chemical additives.

Britain, which has only started to campai
for prevention in the last few years, has seen
slight drop in its heart death rate. It still rem
the highest in the world, killing roughly one person
every three minutes. In Japan and among Eskimos,
where raw fish is a staple diet, heart disease is a fraction
of what it is in most western countries. As soon as
Japanese and Eskimos stop eating traditional food and
become addicted to the same high fat diet of the
Americans and British, however, they too quickly suc-
cumb to heart disease. Japanese communities established
in America, for example, have exactly the same level of
heart disease as the rest of the population.

History also points the finger at modern living and
eating habits as a prime suspect in the heart disease
saga. Records show that only 100 years ago in America
there were no deaths at all per 100,000 population from
heart disease, and it is widely accepted that the first
deaths officially due to heart disease were not recorded
until 1912. By contrast, autopsies (post mortems) on US
soldiers killed in action in Vietnam in the 1970s showed
that half of them had the beginnings of atheroma
(blocked arteries). Their average age was 22. Today in
many western countries children as young as ten are
known to have a level of arterial disease that even adult
ancient Egyptians did not suffer from, according to evidence from 5,000-year-old mummies.

What about other factors?

Bad eating habits are not the only reasons for the development of heart disease but, with stress, are probably
the main ones, although experts will argue. Next come
lack of exercise and being overweight – often precisely

...use of eating and drinking too much of the wrong ...ods and liquids. Other major factors are smoking (although smoking is common in those Mediterranean countries where heart disease is low), and drinking too much alcohol. All, together or in isolation, can end in a heart attack.

As the tables on the following pages show, most of the causes of heart disease are well within the power of the individual to do something about. The basic message is clear: act sooner, before an attack happens, rather than later. Later may be too late.

How to reduce emotional strain

The following is a simple exercise you can try yourself to reduce the main stresses and strains of daily living. Before you get up in the morning make yourself a few basic promises for the day ahead, such as saying:
'Today I will
- have no ill-feelings towards anyone
- accept people for what they are
- not be envious or jealous, arrogant or supercilious
- not get worked up about trivial things
- be friendly and considerate towards everyone
- identify at least one aim or purpose which makes my life worthwhile.'

If you find you can't do this, or fail miserably every time you try even though you'd really like to succeed, it is probably worth seeing a professional therapist for help and support.

Stress and strain

Some stress is necessary and helpful – the sort of stress involved in competitive sport for example – and we can call this 'positive' or 'healthy' stress. But as we saw in the last chapter prolonged mental and emotional strain ('bad stress') can be very definitely unhealthy, and even dangerous. This sort of stress can be handled with a combination of self-help techniques and help from a specialist therapist. Methods include relaxation therapy, meditation, counselling, psychotherapy, hypnotherapy, massage, exercise and yoga (see chapters 8 and 9).

Eating
A guide to sensible and healthy eating is given on pages 62-3 *(figure 6)*. The examples represent most experts' agreed ideas but it is not comprehensive. A 'Mediterranean-style' diet is clearly indicated but you should feel free to add your own choices as long as you see them in terms of low, medium and high risk foods. *As a general rule, foods to be avoided are 'refined' or processed foods and those with lots of fat, sugar and salt.* All will do you damage. Added sugar and salt are simply bad. You do not need either because your body gets all it needs from fresh fruit and vegetables (although it won't get all the nutrients it needs this way – see chapter 9).

- **Salt** is basically a preservative. Its use in modern food processing means most people consume more than 20 times the amount their body really needs, and it raises blood pressure in susceptible people.
- **Sugar** turns to fat if it is not used up as energy, increases the 'stickiness' of blood, raises blood pressure, decreases resistance to stress and can lead to diabetes.
- **Fats** come in different forms and not all are bad. Some can even be beneficial (although all fats are high in calories and can therefore affect your weight - see below). The main types of fat are cholesterol, saturated or animal fat, monounsaturated fat and polyunsaturated fat:
  Cholesterol is a type of blood fat and is essential to the body. As explained in chapter 6 its role is much misunderstood. It is not so much the 'baddie' it is made out to be as the innocent victim.

FOODS	EAT REGULARLY
Cakes, biscuits and desserts	Homemade cakes and biscuits made using low-fat recipes
Cereals and breads	Wholemeal and homemade flour and bread, porridge oats, rice, pasta, breakfast cereals without added sugar and salt
Dairy food and eggs	Skimmed milk, cottage cheese, curd cheese, egg white, low-fat yoghurt, low-fat fromage frais
Drinks and soups	Water, fruit juice, clear soups
Fats and oils	Olive oil (but remember all fats need to be limited)
Fish	Sardines, tuna, salmon, mackerel, trout, white fish, including haddock, cod, plaice (steamed, grilled or baked – *not* fried)
Fruit, vegetables and pulses	Most kinds – fresh, dried, frozen (not canned) – especially alfalfa, garlic, ginger, onions and pineapple. Tofu and other soya products
Meat	Chicken, turkey (both without skin), lean ham
Nuts and seeds	Nuts, except coconut and salted nuts, may be included in vegetarian diets to replace meat Seeds (sunflower, pumpkin, sesame, alfalfa, etc)
Other	Herbs, spices, mustard, cider vinegar, Worcester sauce, low-fat salad dressing
Preserves, spreads and sweets	*None*

Figure 6 Guide to eating and drinking for a healthy heart

EAT IN MODERATION	AVOID ALTOGETHER
Occasional cakes, puddings and biscuits made with polyunsaturated margarine/oil (two or three times a week), ice-cream, jellies, sorbets, skimmed milk puddings	Ready-made cakes and biscuits, cream cakes, dairy cream ice-cream, full-fat milk puddings
Plain semi-sweet biscuits (eg rich tea, digestive), water biscuits, white flour, white bread	Fancy bread and pastries (eg, croissants, brioches), cream crackers
Semi-skimmed milk; medium-fat cheese (such as Edam, Brie, Camembert, Parmesan) not more than three times a week; half-fat cheeses (eg half-fat Cheddar); egg yolks (4 a week maximum)	Full cream milk, cream cheese, most blue cheeses (eg Stilton), full-fat yoghurt, condensed milk, cream, coffee creamers, Cheddar cheese
Alcohol, low-fat drinking chocolate and malted drinks, coffee, tea	Cream soups, full-fat milk drinks and shakes, cream-based drinks
Polyunsaturated margarines and oil (eg safflower oil, corn oil, sunflower oil), linseed (flaxseed) oil, soybean oil, walnut oil, low-fat spreads	Butter, dripping, lard, ghee, margarines not labelled *high in polyunsaturates*, blended vegetable oils
Shellfish (eg lobster, crab, prawns)	Any fish fried in batter, fish roe (eg taramasalata), fish pâté
Chips and roast potatoes cooked in oil marked *high in polyunsaturates* or olive oil (once a fortnight), avocados, olives	Crisps, chips cooked in oil other than olive oil or oil marked *high in polyunsaturates*
Lean cuts of beef, pork, lamb, lean bacon (unsmoked), lean mince, liver, kidney, meat paste (Not more than three times a week)	Visible fat on meat; sausages, pâté, duck, salami, meat pies and pasties, pork pies
Salted nuts	Coconut
Low-calorie salad cream and mayonnaise, French dressing made with polyunsaturated or olive oil	Salad cream, mayonnaise, creamy dressings
Jam, marmalade, honey, peanut butter	Chocolates, toffees, fudge, mincemeat containing suet, chocolate spread, sugar, all sweets and confectionery

Saturated fat is generally thought to be the main fat bad guy. Found in animal foods like red meat and dairy products, it is commonly also called 'animal fat' and has been linked to raised blood cholesterol.

Monounsaturated fat is good for you. It is found in olive oil but is only beneficial if you buy the oil 'cold-pressed'. Olive oil extracted using heat is changed and becomes harmful. Bottles should be labelled 'extra virgin cold-pressed'.

Polyunsaturated fat is also good for you, in moderation. It is found in vegetable oils, like corn oil, sunflower and safflower oil, and in oily fish like tuna and sardines as well as in some margarines (but avoid margarines, and any foods, containing hydrogenated or processed fat which is a known 'villain').

Examples of foods which are unhealthily high in saturated fats are pork sausages, pork pies, hamburgers, french fries, samosa, full-fat milk, cream cheese, cheddar cheese, butter, cheesecake, chocolate and biscuits (cookies). Low-fat diet foods are baked and boiled potatoes, poached fish, yoghurt, skimmed milk, ham and cottage cheese.

The more fresh fruit and vegetables you eat the better. Foods like lentils, beans, peas and oats contain a type of dietary fibre which is good for the blood, and in the case of a food like alfalfa there is even some evidence it reverses atheroma. But you don't have to be a vegetarian to be healthy and avoid heart disease. Fish, poultry and even lean meat are relatively low in fat (provided you cut off all the obvious fat, including chicken and turkey skin) and contain good nutrients. Buy organic to avoid meat with growth hormones and antibiotics.

When it comes to cooking, avoid frying as much as possible in favour of grilling, steaming, poaching or roasting without adding fat. Avoid ready-made meals and indeed as much processed, refined and tinned food as possible: they are usually high in fat, salt and sugar as well as many sorts of undesirable chemical additives, colourings and preservatives (such as the dangerous *monosodium glutamate*). Always read labels and, if necessary, ask the store manager for more explanation.

Teeth and the heart

If you know you have heart disease it is important to visit a dentist regularly and keep teeth and gums healthy. Poor dental hygiene can lead to a dangerous heart condition known as *infective endocarditis*. Bacteria enter the bloodstream through bleeding gums and cause inflammation of the heart valves. It is particularly dangerous for people who already have defective or artificial valves. Good and regular brushing with a proper toothpaste and an occasional massage of the gums with a finger is the best prevention.

Weight

Figure 7 gives an indication of what your weight should be for your height. Although it shows it is possible to be underweight this is rare in western societies where people generally eat far more than they really need to stay healthy. Usually the leaner people are the fitter they are but overweight verging on obesity is common in the industrial world – and puts sufferers at high risk of heart disease. *More than half of those who are overweight are likely to die of heart disease.*

According to Russian obesity expert Dr Tamara Voronina, who runs a specialist clinic in London: 'Obesity is not merely a cosmetic problem but a serious illness. Even a small weight excess changes the body's metabolism, leads to an increase in blood cholesterol, promotes ageing and results in ischaemic heart disease, hypertension (high blood pressure), diabetes and gall bladder abnormalities. There is also an increased risk of more dramatic problems such as carcinomas (cancer) of the colon, rectum and prostate in men, and of the breast, uterus, ovaries and cervix in women. The lowest mortality risk is associated with a body weight 5-15 per cent below the European average. Thus even a small increase in body weight is potentially life-threatening.'

Losing weight safely and effectively is a matter of burning up more energy (calories) than you generate. Energy comes mostly from what we eat and drink (and from the air we breathe) so the only effective way to lose weight is to eat less. A good weight loss programme is one which is as 'natural' as possible (so don't take appetite-suppressants such as *fenfluoramine* and *mazindol* or thyroid hormones which excite the metabolism), makes sure you lose weight gradually but regularly within the limits of your height and weight (your natural 'mass') and does not see the weight go back on when you stop. Controlled fasting for limited periods (longer than 24 hours) under proper supervision – not the same as crash-dieting – is a recognized therapeutic approach described in more detail in chapter 9.

Weight-loss programmes are everywhere these days. The best advice is to choose a diet in which you are still eating real, healthy food – not food substitutes or powders. The Pritkin Diet is an ultra low-fat 'real food' diet which has found some fame in America through the work of Dr Ornish but there are many others. The Hay Diet, the Wright Diet, the 'Plus-Minus' Diet and Michio Kushi's 'Macrobiotic Diet' are all well known diets that make use of the principle of 'food combining' widely followed in the Orient and with a well-reported track record of success. Remember, though, dieting usually causes the body's metabolism to slow down and adjust to less food. It is important, therefore, to diet *and exercise* for maximum effect.

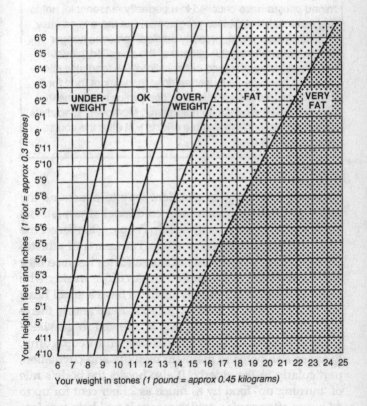

Figure 7 Are you the right height for your weight?
By courtesy of the British Heart Foundation

Acupuncture can take away hunger pangs

Probably the hardest part of dieting for anyone who is very overweight is overcoming hunger pangs. A person who overeats has a stretched stomach and it does not take kindly to being asked to remain empty while it slowly contracts to its proper size. And overeating, especially 'comfort-eating', is an ingrained habit as hard to break as any other. Hunger pangs are probably the main reason why many quite determined people have chucked in a perfectly reasonable, not to say essential, weight-loss programme. But there is an easy answer: Acupuncture, properly applied, removes hunger pangs by stimulating the release of the so-called 'pleasure hormones' endorphin and encephalin which food also stimulates. So because acupuncture does the work of food for it your stomach does not miss the food (which means neither do you!) and the pangs do not appear. Moreover, specialists in the technique claim that the effects last after the course of acupuncture is over.

Exercise

Exercise is not only an excellent way to overcome the major problem of mental and emotional strain (stress) but it is also vital for heart health. People often forget the heart is a muscle, made to work. The hearts of athletes are often larger than those of non-athletes because they are worked hard and kept in trim. An office worker who takes no exercise is not only likely to have a small heart but also one that is 'flabby'. It lacks 'tone' and is therefore less efficient. A heart that is allowed to get 'lazy' finds it harder to fight off disease and keep going. Exercise also helps to maintain mobility and circulation, particularly in the elderly. It also boosts the body's rate of 'burning up' food by as much as 25 per cent for up to 48 hours afterwards – which means it will help you lose weight more quickly too.

The purpose of exercise is to get fit and that means to get the heart fit. Fitness means having suppleness, strength and stamina. Experts say that to achieve minimum fitness you should exert yourself for at least 20 minutes three or four times a week. That means working up a good 'sweat' by walking, climbing, jogging, swimming, cycling or whatever it takes to make you breathe more heavily and take in more oxygen (which is what the word 'aerobic' means). The important thing is to keep your pulse rate up for a full 20 minutes. This will also help slim you down. But be careful to moderate your exercise level against your pulse rate. You should not let your pulse go above a figure 60-80 per cent of 220 less your age. It is not the purpose of this book to give aerobic exercises but exercises for suppleness are a feature of yoga (see chapter 9). Remember, fitness can't be stored – it has to be worked at all the time.

How fit are you?

You will know if you need to do something about your physical fitness if you answer 'yes' to all or even most of the following questions:

- Do you get out of breath fairly quickly walking up a slope?
- Do your legs ache or feel weak after you've climbed stairs?
- Do you find it difficult to bend down to tie shoelaces or put on socks or tights?
- Do you find it difficult to reach behind your head to pull off a jumper or comb your hair?
- Do you find it difficult to get out of a bath or armchair?

Caution Sudden strenuous exercise by very obese people or people over 55 who have done no exercise for many years is dangerous and can lead to a heart attack. Work into it gradually – but get a proper medical checkup first.

Drinking

Some alcohol is not harmful and indeed may even be beneficial. There is evidence, for example, that red wine made from Merlot grapes (such as the claret 'St Emilion') contains antioxidant chemicals called phenolic compounds which help prevent atherosclerosis. But moderation in all things is the key and too much alcohol is very definitely harmful. The table below shows the safe levels for both men and women. The same applies to both tea and coffee: there is no evidence that either is very harmful if drunk in moderation (which means no more than 3-4 cups a day). But remember, no sugar or sweetener!

Alcohol consumption guide		
	Maximum level	**Dangerous level**
Women	14 units a week	Over 35 units a week
Men	21 units a week	Over 50 units a week
1 unit = 1 ordinary glass of wine/1 ordinary measure of spirit/1 glass (or half-a-pint) of beer.		

How to use this information

It requires a fairly high degree of self-discipline to change all those many bad habits that most of us have got pretty used to by the time it comes round to having to change it all. Change, however, is very definitely the name of the game if heart disease is not to be allowed either to develop or get worse, and it is even more important if you want to reverse it. Dean Ornish, the US medical 'guru' of natural ways to beat heart disease, insists it is only those who want to change, and make a commited effort to change, who get better. For the rest, he says, 'I don't hesitate to use drugs and surgery.'

We know a lot about avoiding heart disease and this knowledge is the most important weapon we have. The body has a natural built-in ability to balance itself out. It is called *homoeostasis* (from Greek words meaning 'self-regulation'). In other words the body will cure itself of almost anything given half a chance. Following a healthy diet, taking exercise and learning to relax will *on their own* – as Dean Ornish has proved – go a long way to halting the effects of atherosclerosis (clogging of arteries) and even reversing them altogether. Diet, exercise and relaxation are, indeed, the three most natural of the natural ways to treat heart disease.

The first step in any self-help programme is to make the basic decision to take responsibility for your own health. Fortunately, in the case of heart disease, there is a great deal you can do for yourself by yourself without needing to consult a doctor or therapist at all.

For example, if you suffer from angina (heart pain) you may be persuaded that what you need is an immediate bypass operation. But unless there are very good reasons why you should have an immediate bypass – in which case make sure the reasons are given to you and that you understand and accept them – consider that you may be able to cure yourself by the various methods described in this book. An operation may be the very last thing you need or should have. So be prepared to stand up for yourself and question closely any doctor who is keen to rush you straight off to the operating table.

The basic rules of self-help

Almost everyone is agreed on the basic rules of self-help for heart disease and even though they are all basically very obvious and based on common-sense it is still surprising how many people ignore them. They are:

● learn how to handle your stress levels and take time to relax (see chapter 8 for therapies that can help)

- control what you eat and drink. For example,
  - drink plenty of good, clean water (at least 2 litres a day),
  - avoid sugar, salt, saturated fats and processed food,
  - eat as little as possible of dairy products (especially cow's milk and cheese), but
  - eat plenty of fresh fruit and vegetables, fish and fibre,
  - drink alcohol in moderation (no more than 3 units of alcohol a day for men, 2 for women),
- take regular exercise (at least 20 minutes three times a week),
- get down to (or make sure you stick at) your 'ideal' weight,
- don't smoke (or no more than two or three a day).

Making out a health programme for yourself

So knowing this what can you do about it? The first thing you can do is to sit down and start to take a cool, hard, honest look at yourself and your lifestyle. Try the following simple exercise: Take a sheet of paper and a pen and sit down somewhere comfortable with a healthy glass of mineral water. Now draw three columns on your piece of paper and head them, from left to right, 'What I do', 'What I should do' and 'What I need to do'. Down the left hand side write the main risk factors, like this:

	What I do	What I should do	What I need to do
Stress factors	List problems	Ideals	Targets
Eating habits	List regular foods	Ideals	Targets
Exercise habits	How much exercise?	Ideals	Targets
Weight	Existing weight	Ideal	Target
Smoking habits	How many a day?	Ideal	Target
Drinking habits	How much a day?	Ideal	Target

In the first 'What I do' column write down what you do as honestly as you can (no one is going to see it except you after all!). Now, using the information in this book, decide what your 'ideal' lifestyle should be to be healthy and write it down in the second 'What I should do' column. That is your ideal. Finally compare the two columns and in the third 'What I need to do' column write down what you need to do to reach the ideal. That is your target. It is now up to you to decide if you are going to go for it or not, and how you are going to do it.

Let's assume you've decided to go for it. A useful next step for most people, particularly those with good old human weaknesses like most of us, is to make out a programme for yourself.

The first thing to do is to decide priorities: what do you think you can cope with, and when? For example, you may think you can cut down on alcohol right away but cutting out cigarettes is going to be a real struggle. So for week one you can probably write down your alcohol target (21 units a week if you're a man, 14 if you're a woman) from day one. But you will probably have to try and phase out smoking over a longer period so decide if you can cut down by, say, a quarter the first week (from, say, 20 to 15 cigarettes a day), a half the next and so on until you've stopped altogether. The idea is to hit your target *eventually* even if it takes weeks. You must decide you want to do it and have the will-power to do it. It's your health, don't forget, and no one can do it but you – although there are natural therapies than can help you. Both acupuncture and hypnosis, for example, can help you stop smoking.

Working out what to do with stress factors may be the hardest but the important point here is not to hold anything back. This is an exercise for you and no one else so let it all go. Put down in column one everything you can think of that drives you crazy – from the job, the kids, the car, the neighbours, the house, whatever. It may be the solution is easier than you think. Changing your job, moving somewhere more more congenial or taking a holiday can often make a huge difference on their own. Facing the prospect of change is often the hardest part of change.

Of course it may mean changing yourself (if you're a man this is quite likely!) and that's not so easy. Or it may be that the whole thing is just too much to handle. Perhaps you have symptoms of heart disease already and are afraid. You don't know where to start or even how. If any of this applies to you then you need help.

The most obvious source of help is your own immediate family and friends. Talk to them and tell them you would like support in your attempts to improve your health and well-being. Ask them to help you stop having those extra drinks and cigarettes, to encourage you to eat sensibly and take exercise – even to share the experience and do the programme with you. But sometimes this is not easy to achieve, and even if it is the support you need is simply not forthcoming. It is at this point you may need to turn to a specialist in natural medicine. In the second half of the book we'll look at the options available.

CHAPTER 6

Conventional treatments and procedures

What your doctor is likely to say

If you've decided that despite your best efforts you really aren't getting any better, or that you can't find the way or the will to do things for yourself, you have the choice of two routes in seeking professional help: the conventional route or the route of natural therapy. In this chapter we'll cover the conventional route.

The conventional way to treat arterial disease is by drugs and surgery. Before treatment will come the tests or diagnosis. Most doctors have been trained to follow more or less the same procedure whether you have gone to them for a general check-up or a specific problem such as angina. They will:

- weigh and measure you
- take your blood pressure
- do blood and urine tests, and (sometimes)
- take an electrocardiogram (ECG) reading.

They will be looking to see, basically, if you are too heavy for your height and bone structure, if your blood pressure is too high, if you have any abnormal heart rhythms, if you are diabetic, and finally if you have high cholesterol levels. The results of these tests will determine your treatment.

Check your diagnosis

Conventional treatment for heart and arterial disease involves the prescription of drugs in the early stages, but if the disease starts to show symptoms the doctor might consider serious surgery is the next step. So the most important thing to decide next is to be as sure as you can be that you have been correctly diagnosed. Even experienced doctors do not always apply as much knowledge as they should to the three vital tests of blood pressure, cholesterol level and ECG.

Older patients, for example, can sometimes be wrongly diagnosed as having blood pressure that is too high by the arm cuff technique of reading pressure when in fact it is perfectly normal and healthy for their age. The stiffness in their arteries due to age leads to an over-reading known as 'pseudo-hypertension'. Also the older we get the less significant the lower (diastolic) reading over the higher (systolic). Diastolic pressure levels out over the age of around 60 but systolic continues to increase. As a very rough-and-ready rule, systolic should not be more than your age plus 100. Thus a man of 80 with a reading of 160 (systolic) over 95 or even 100 (diastolic) – usually written 160/100 – is likely to have what can be regarded as perfectly normal blood pressure while that same reading in a man of 40 or even 50 would be a cause for some alarm, and immediate treatment.

Pay particular attention to the relevance and weight the doctor gives to your blood cholesterol reading. As we have already seen, cholesterol is not as all-powerfully significant as it is being claimed and you should remain unimpressed if the doctor quickly starts talking about drugs on the basis of readings that may give a misleading idea of your real blood health (see chapter 4).

ECG readings also can be misleading, depending not only on who has done the reading but also on whether

Check your doctor's approach

Medicine generally moves only slowly with the times and new thinking and developments can take as long as a generation to become standard practice. Not all doctors will be unsympathetic to the natural or 'holistic' approaches in this book and there is an easy way to find out if your doctor is holistic or not. Some 'warning signs' may help you.

Prevention is better than cure and any sympathetic doctor's first priority is always going to be to get you to change your lifestyle to reduce your chances of developing arterial disease. Even if you know you already have affected arteries lifestyle changes can be beneficial so treatment should start with advice on what changes to make. Since there is a fairly broad consensus on this the advice is likely to follow more or less the guidelines already outlined in previous chapters, including how to control your stress levels and your general emotional and psychological state.

The first warning sign is if he or she fails to give such advice, or, worse, opposes it if you suggest it yourself.

The second warning sign is if your doctor tells you that arterial disease is inevitable. If he or she says or even implies it is a natural and unavoidable part of growing old and there is nothing to it but resigning yourself to progressive infirmity fed by unpleasant drugs with nasty side-effects and, eventually, surgery, beware! It is not true and you should not believe it, still less accept it.

The third warning sign is if you are not taken into the doctor's confidence about the treatments he or she wants to give you. A good doctor should explain and discuss all the options and possible side-effects and should seek your opinion. Doctors don't always know and if they know they don't always say, but treatment should be a partnership. Whose body, mind and soul is it anyway?

If any of the above warning signs flash up you should think seriously about continuing treatment with this particular doctor.

the test was a 'resting' ECG or an 'exercise' or 'stress' ECG in which your heartbeat is measured during exercise. Resting ECGs, especially, are so inaccurate and inconclusive that as many as 30 per cent of people with actual heart disease produce a 'normal' ECG reading (known as a 'false negative') while between 20-50 per cent of those with no heart disease show a positive reading ('false positive').

Drug treatments

When doctors say they are going to give you 'pills for your heart' they usually mean they are going to use drugs to treat either high blood pressure or high blood cholesterol or both. Both are considered serious risk factors and suitable for drug therapy. The important thing for you to decide is if you really want to be committed to long-term drug use for conditions that can be treated by non-drug means and may not even need drugs at all. In the case of drugs for both blood pressure and high cholesterol there is growing evidence that they may actually cause more harm than good.

Remember that though drugs have been subjected to scientific tests to confirm their efficacy they also have side-effects. The reason they have been licensed for release is because they have passed the so-called 'risk-benefit ratio' test. This means simply that experts have decided that their benefits outweigh their disadvantages. This applies to all drugs and is the reason to be very careful about the use of synthetic drugs generally. There are almost always disadvantages or side-effects for many people and 'experts' do not always get it right any more than they can necessarily be relied upon to be free of the taint of vested interest in the outcome. Since the majority of drugs are tested in secret and the results held in secret (because they are the work of competing commercial companies) there is no way of knowing how 'straight' those behind them have been. Outcomes are frequently decided in advance and there is evidence from 'defectors' from the medical research industry to suggest that profit more than the desire to heal is often the main motive.

Drugs for treating high blood pressure

These drugs fall into four categories: ACE inhibitors, beta-blockers, diuretics, and calcium antagonists.

- **ACE inhibitors** (medical names include *captopril, cilazapril, enalapril, lisinopril, perindopril*) work by widening the body's blood vessels to improve blood flow. The most common side-effects are dizziness when starting the drug and severe 'dry' coughing, but they can also cause diarrhoea, headache, nausea, rash, loss of taste and kidney failure. They do not work well in Afro-Caribbean people.
- **Beta-blockers** (*atenolol , bisoprolol, metaprolol, celiprolol, labetalol, oxprenolol, propranolol*) are thought to act by slowing down the heart rate and making the heart pump better. Common side-effects are cold fingers and toes and a feeling of 'slowing down', but they have also produced sleep and breathing problems, dry eyes and rash. Also not so effective in Afro-Caribbeans.
- **Diuretics** (*bendrofluazide, cyclopenthiazide, hydrochlor-thiazide, hydroflumethiazide, methylclothiazide, polythi-azide*) help the heart work more efficiently by increasing the amount of water the body loses, which in turn reduces the amount of blood in the body. Known side-effects, especially in high doses, are rashes, dizziness, headaches, fatigue, confusion, acute gout and impotence. They also remove essential

potassium from the blood, increase blood fats (especially cholesterol) and uric acid, and produce intolerance to glucose.

- **Calcium antagonists** (*amlodipine, felodipine, isradipine, nicardipine, nifedipine*) inhibit the action of muscles to stop them squeezing the blood vessels. Side-effects include dizziness, flushing, headaches, palpitations, nausea, rashes and swollen ankles. Two particular classes, *verapamil* and *diltiazem*, can cause heart failure.

It's difficult to stop taking blood pressure drugs once you've started (though not impossible) so before you commit yourself check your doctor has taken into account all the right factors such as your age, family history, other risk factors and, most important of all, that you have done all you can to reduce your blood pressure naturally (see chapter 5).

Drugs for treating high blood cholesterol

These drugs are of four types: bile acid sequestrants, nicotinic and isobutyric acid derivatives, and hydroxy-methylglutaryl coenzyme A (HMG CoA) reductase inhibitors.

- **Bile acid sequestrants** (examples *cholestyramine* and *colestipol*) work by decreasing the level of cholesterol in the blood by interfering with the way the bile acid-cholesterol balance is handled by the liver. *Cholestyramine*, described by one doctor as 'an unpleasant drug, not dissimilar to swallowing a mouthful of sand before each meal', can cause dyspepsia, flatulence, constipation and heartburn. A variant is *probucol* whose action doctors admit they do not understand and which seems to cause as much harm as good. Side-effects include diarrhoea and upset stomach.

- **Nicotinic acid derivatives** (*nicofuranose, acipimox*) act on the liver and blood vessels to lower both cholesterol and triglyceride levels in the blood by interfering with cholesterol production in the liver and increasing cholesterol excretion. Nicotinic acid itself produces intense flushing and headaches. Other side-effects are rash, upset stomach and 'feeling low'.

- **Isobutyric acid derivatives** (*bezafibrate, cipofibrate, clofibrate, fenofibrate, gemfibrozil*) also work by reducing blood cholesterol and triglycerides by interfering with the way the liver works and increasing excretion via the gut through the gall bladder. One of the most important side-effects is the risk of gallstones. Others include upset stomach, rash, myalgia, headache, fatigue, vertigo, impotence, cramps, dizziness, blurred vision, 'painful extremities', hair loss and drowsiness.

- **HMG CoA reductase inhibitors** (*pravastatin, simvastatin*) are the latest generation of cholesterol-lowering drugs and represent a 'last-ditch' approach for people with high cholesterol levels which have not responded to other drugs. They act by blocking the production of cholesterol in the liver and increasing excretion and are claimed to reduce LDL ('bad') -cholesterol levels in the blood by up to 40 per cent. Side-effects, however, include rash, myalgia, headache, chest pain, nausea, vomiting, diarrhoea, fatigue, constipation, flatulence, dyspepsia, stomach pain and 'feeling weak'.

Accepting drug treatment for high blood pressure and high blood cholesterol is a very serious step. Once you start it is hard to stop because your body comes to rely on the drugs, so blood pressure and cholesterol are likely to go up when you stop. Also coming off drugs can take real effort and commitment. It is therefore important to decide if there is absolutely *no other alternative* before you go ahead. You should be quite sure you

'Semi-conventional' drug treatments

Aware of the short-comings of drugs but unaware of the gentler alternatives, doctors are recommending two drug treatments that are not generally well known for heart disease:

● **Aspirin**, derived originally from the plant compound salicin found in willow and meadowsweet, is an anticoagulant as well as a pain-killer (analgesic). That means it acts as a thinning agent on the blood and so helps it to flow better. It is taken in tablet form in the same way as for a headache (half a tablet, between 75-325mg, every morning is routinely recommended to prevent heart attack) but can also be given as an emergency treatment during or after a heart attack by injection. There can be side-effects, however, the main ones being heartburn, stomach pain and bleeding (resulting in blood in the stools), nausea and vomiting. In January 1994 a survey of the research to date concluded that because of these side-effects aspirin should *not* be taken routinely for prevention. It should only be taken if you already have heart disease or have had a heart attack, when the benefits may outweigh the risks.

● **Hormone Replacement Therapy (HRT)** is used to top up or replace the hormones oestrogen and progesterone which a woman does not produce in the same quantity after the menopause (cessation of monthly periods). Oestrogen is believed to be one of the main reasons younger women have much lower levels of heart disease than men. HRT is considered essential for women who have had a hysterectomy (removal of the womb). It is given usually in tablet form but also as an implant, a plaster 'patch' and a vaginal cream. It is claimed to be useful against heart disease – and also osteoporosis (brittle bones, particularly in elderly women) – if taken on a long-term basis and if you are in the groups considered at high risk (see chapter 1). However short-term side-effects can include vomiting, abdominal cramps, bloating and jaundice, and long-term use – particularly of oestrogen-only forms – can lead to drug dependency, breast cancer, cancer of the womb lining and to periods returning in your sixties and seventies.

have been thoroughly and properly diagnosed and that you have done your utmost to bring down your levels naturally. Remember that doctors are only human and many a good but hard-pressed and harrassed doctor will prescribe drugs because it is the easiest and quickest thing to do. Most drugs are over-prescribed very much because of this pressure on doctors. The only real beneficiaries in this situation are the makers of the drugs, the pharmaceutical industry.`

Note For people with very high blood pressure and very high blood fats, especially those with an inherited tendency like *familial hyperlipidaemia* (see chapter 1), drugs may be the only option. But in such cases the natural ways can still help conventional treatments work better and damage you less.

Surgery: the final step

A doctor who persuades you onto the moving walkway of conventional drug treatment is a doctor who probably sees surgery as the next, and final, step. From simple diagnostic tests and drugs you will be moved to exploratory 'high-tech' surgery such as coronary angiography and full-scale operations such as bypass surgery or balloon angioplasty. These techniques are major surgical interventions, they are risky, painful and imperfect and none is a cure. You should be told this, and if you are not it is as well you know. Let's take a closer look at them.

Angiography

Angiography (or arteriography) is not a treatment so much as a diagnostic technique. It involves threading a catheter (small tube) into the heart and its arteries and injecting a special dye into them so an x-ray picture can be taken. The picture is supposed to show up any blockages in the arteries. It is generally regarded by doctors as the 'gold standard' in judging the extent and severity of coronary artery disease and so to decide if surgery is necessary. But it is under increasing attack for being inaccurate, overused and dangerous. In 1992 the *Journal of the American Medical Association* reported a US study that found that only four per cent of patients advised to have angiography really needed one – and 4,500 patients had actually died as a direct result of the procedure. But even if you don't die the process can cause nausea, anxiety and rapid heart-beat.

'The angiogram is one of the most inaccurate tests in modern medicine', American health campaigner Dr Julian Whittaker has said. 'Comparisons of angiogram readings and actual measurements of blood-flow through arteries have proven that the angiogram is so inaccurate as to be virtually useless.' Nevertheless it remains the most important method by which doctors the world over decide if someone is to have heart surgery or not. So what of the surgery?

Surgery is the end of the line in conventional medical treatment, the call at the 'last chance' saloon. There are two methods currently competing for favour: bypass surgery and angioplasty.

Bypass surgery

Bypass surgery, or more correctly *coronary artery bypass graft* (CABG), is the older of the two treatments having been introduced in the late 1960s and it is now regarded as a routine operation to such an extent that it is almost automatic for people with heart disease in the USA where more than 300,000 operations a year are carried out. The technique involves 'bypassing' blocked arteries on the surface of the heart by grafting in clean veins from another part of the body, usually the leg. The veins are stripped out of the leg and attached to the heart around the blocked artery. The operation, which involves the chest being opened up for what has become known as 'open-heart' surgery, is dangerous and painful. *Most important of all it is not a cure.* It is effective for only so long: an average of 5-7.5 years, according to the latest British research, but seldom more than 10-12 years.

A Canadian doctor, Dr Zigurts Strauts from Vancouver, claimed in a US newsletter for doctors in 1992 that in America as many as one in every 20 people going in for the operation do not leave the operating room alive, one in every five suffer from some form of brain damage, and among other reported complications have been several cases of kidney failure.

Problems in heart surgery

More mental and emotional trauma, or psychological disturbance, is felt after heart surgery than any other type of surgery. It is commonly caused by one, or all, of the following:

- Tiny blood clots formed in the heart-lung machine used during the surgery enter the body and lodge in the brain. The mental confusion they cause is usually temporary but they can cause permanent brain damage.
- 'Deadening' drugs such as *scopolamine* and *droperidol* used by anaesthetists to reduce the stress of the operation can cause a sense of unreality and affect memory.
- Some anaesthetics knock you out for the operation but don't shut down your sense of hearing – so your brain can recall the sounds of the operation afterwards, sometimes leading to nightmares.

Angioplasty

Angioplasty, or 'balloon angioplasty', was introduced in 1977 as a less invasive alternative to bypass surgery. Instead of arteries being replaced or bypassed by opening up the chest wall surgeons thread a tube into the blocked or partially blocked arteries and force them open by inflating a tiny balloon in the end of the tube and using it like a pipe-cleaner. The tube is usually fed into the body through the large arteries in the groin that lead straight to the heart *(see figure 3)*. Doctors call this technique *percutaneous transluminal coronary angioplasty* (PTCA) and in America, especially, it has become so popular it has replaced bypass as the surgeons' treatment of choice for blocked arteries. But it, too, is now under attack for being dangerous, short-term and ineffective. Dr Strauts claimed that in America about two per cent of patients routinely do not survive the operation and in California the figure one year was nearly five per cent. Moreover, the operation is seldom effective for more than about two years and frequently for as little as six months or less.

US cardiologist Dr Thomas Graboy, who carried out a special study of the practice in 1992, found that half of all angioplasties performed in the USA were unnecessary. Attacking the enthusiasm for both bypass surgery and angioplasty he said: 'Some of the hoopla for costly procedures [bypass surgery and angioplasty] are not driven by rigorous medical indications but are propelled by vested economic interests.' It was his way of saying that some US heart surgeons earn in excess of $1 million a year carrying out such procedures, and the drugs companies even more, so small wonder they are popular – with the surgeons and drugs companies!

Bypass and angioplasty compared
In Britain the first major trial comparing bypass with angioplasty as a treatment for angina reported its halfway stage findings in the leading medical journal the *Lancet* in March 1993. Press coverage concentrated on the fact that bypass surgery came out ahead as being more

effective. In fact neither procedure won many honours.
A table published afterwards by the prestigious British
Heart Foundation, which provides heavy financial support for both drug therapy and surgery as the treatments
of choice for heart disease, showed that both surgical
procedures had disadvantages which far outweighed the
advantages.

	Advantages	Disadvantages
Bypass surgery	● Greater relief.	● In hospital for over a week.
	● Medication less likely after.	● Less active after a month.
		● Off work for 2-3 months.
		● More short-term discomfort.
Angioplasty	● In hospital 2-3 days.	● Angina returns in a third of patients within 6 months.
	● Back to work sooner.	● Further investigation four times more common afterwards.
		● Repeat treatment needed within 2 years in a third of patients.
		● Medication more likely afterwards.

In summary

Conventional medicine tends to see heart disease as preventable and therefore 'naturally' treatable – up to a
point. Beyond that point, which is whenever any of the
'risk factors' such as high blood pressure and high

cholesterol show no signs of shifting in the right direction, doctors start to want to intervene – and that means drugs probably followed by surgery. They are not, by and large, too slow in wanting to put people on drugs and as quick, more often than not, in pushing them forward for major surgery. The problem is that in the process they may be ignoring a safe, gentle and effective intermediate stage of treatment that could, and in many cases will, remove the need for the highly risky, traumatic and worrying 'emergency' final stage of drugs and surgery altogether.

Of course it is true that conventional medicine is coming up with new ideas for the diagnosis and treatment of heart and arterial disease all the time but it is equally true that these new ideas – and each of them would probably fill a book on its own – are simply an extension of existing procedures, either better and more powerful drugs or cleverer and more sophisticated surgical techniques. None of them asks the basic question of whether there is a need for either drugs or surgery in the first place, and whether anything can be done before resorting to either. They do not, in other words, ask what can be done at the *intermediate* level.

What treatments are available at the intermediate level? There are many and they are almost all those therapies and approaches that have come to be known as 'natural'.

CHAPTER 7

The natural therapies and heart disease

Introducing the 'gentle alternatives'

If you've decided you don't want to go down the conventional medical route because the idea of powerful synthetic drugs with side-effects and surgery worries you, first of all don't worry. What you are feeling is quite normal. Most people, sometimes those very people who put the sternest face to the world and you think must be as strong as an ox, are unable to see the wood for the trees when it comes to their own health and are just as frightened of therapists with their white coats, different language and strange ways as you are.

Also, if you'd still rather see a doctor, there are fortunately more and more doctors these days who understand and agree with your reservations about modern medicine and are prepared at least to try something different. There are any number of ways of treating heart disease effectively that don't involve either drugs or surgery and the better doctors are becoming familiar with them.

But if you know your family doctor is not one of the enlightened and you have decided you would definitely prefer natural therapy, or you have been recommended a good local practitioner of natural therapy, what can you expect? And how can they help?

Natural therapies useful for heart disease

It will be as much a surprise to many doctors as it may be to you that the list of natural therapies useful in treating heart disease is long (though more and more doctors, particularly the younger ones, are rapidly coming round to the benefits of softer, gentler treatments for much the same reasons you are probably reading this book).

Natural therapies fall very roughly into two types: **psychological therapies** and **physical therapies**. Psychological therapies are aimed at treating your mental and emotional condition whereas physical therapies treat your physical state. However many natural therapies fall into both categories. The list opposite shows, in alphabetical order, the therapies useful in heart disease in the category that is most obvious from their method of working. For example, chiropractic and osteopathy are very obviously physical therapy as 'hands-on' approaches whereas hypnotherapy and psychotherapy are not. Yoga and massage, on the other hand, though they involve physical movement and touch also have a powerful psychological purpose.

Why go to a natural therapist?

A natural health practitioner is, or should be, someone who understands not only you and your problem but is also familiar with the host of safe and gentle treatments that do not involve your being either filled with unpleasant drugs or operated on, and who is prepared to give you plenty of time to explore these options. This person may be a doctor but is just as likely to be a non-medical practitioner of natural, holistic, alternative or complementary therapies (different people favour different descriptions but basically we are talking about the same thing: practitioners who practice what official medicine

PSYCHOLOGICAL THERAPIES	PHYSICAL THERAPIES
Acupuncture/Acupressure (Including Shiatsu)	Acupuncture/Acupressure (Including Shiatsu)
*Aromatherapy	*Alexander Technique
*Art therapy	*Aromatherapy
*Biofeedback	Ayurvedic medicine
*Colour & light therapy	(traditional Indian medicine)
COUNSELLING	CHELATION THERAPY
*Crystal therapy/Electro-crystal therapy	Chiropractic/McTimoney Chiropractic
*Dance & movement therapy	Colon cleansing/Colonic irrigation
*Flower remedies	Cranial osteopathy/Cranio-
*Gem therapy	sacral therapy
Healing/Faith healing/Spiritual healing	*Crystal therapy/Electro-crystal therapy
*Homoeopathy	
HYPNOTHERAPY/HYPNOSIS	*HERBALISM/TRADITIONAL CHINESE MEDICINE
*MASSAGE	
*MEDITATION/Visualization/ Autogenics/ Auto-suggestion	*HYDROTHERAPY
	*MASSAGE
	*NATUROPATHY (Nature Cure/ Natural Hygiene)
*Music & sound therapy	
*Polarity therapy	*NUTRITIONAL THERAPY
PSYCHOTHERAPY/ PSYCHOLOGY (Humanistic Psychology, Transpersonal Psychology etc)	Osteopathy
	Oxygen therapy (hyperbaric oxygen/ hypoxia therapy)
	Radionics
*Reflexology/Zone therapy	*Reflexology/Zone therapy
Vacuflex therapy	Vacuflex therapy
*YOGA	*YOGA

*The starred therapies (*) are those you can do for yourself (self-help) after some initial training. The rest need the services of a trained practitioner. CAPITALS indicate a therapy with proven benefit or strong anecdotal (case history or hearsay) evidence in its favour in heart disease. **Bold** type indicates the therapy is widely known and used.*

likes to call non-conventional or unorthodox medical techniques to treat disease).

People often turn to a natural therapist as a last resort. They have tried the conventional route and it hasn't worked. For whatever reason – and it may be because their problem was not helped or, sadly, perhaps even made worse – their needs haven't been met. An official report in Israel in 1991 concluded that people there were turning in growing numbers to natural medicine for exactly the same reasons they are turning to it the world over: that is, a concern, even outright disillusionment, over an increasingly specialized and rigid medical profession that is slow to respond not only to the fast-changing nature and incidence of disease in a safe and gentle way – preferring synthetic substances and high technology over 'natural' approaches – but also to the public's growing demand for greater freedom of choice in healthcare and a say in how they are treated.

Whatever the reasons people go to practitioners of natural therapy they seem to get a high level of satisfaction when they do. In Britain, for example, where no therapist is legally required to train to practice non-medical therapy, surveys in recent years have consistently shown satisfaction levels between 60-80 per cent. So who are these therapists and what is it about them that appeals so much? What is natural therapy and most important of all, how do you find the right practitioner?

What is natural therapy?

There is a quite a discussion (not to say argument , even among natural therapists themselves) about whether all natural therapies operate under one common idea or principle. The British Medical Association, in a report it published in June 1993, said they did not – that the natural therapies were a mish-mash of different styles and techniques with nothing in common at all. But the BMA was surprisingly misinformed. The natural approaches all understand, accept and operate under the following principles:

- The body has a natural ability to heal and regulate itself.
- The human being is not simply a physical machine, like a car, but a subtle and complex blend of body, mind and emotions (or spirit or soul as some prefer to call it) and that all or any of these factors may cause or contribute to problems of health. In other words, that every individual is not a random collection of moving parts but a fully integrated 'whole'. (The term 'holistic medicine' has been coined to describe treating the individual as a 'whole being' composed of body, mind and spirit.)
- Environmental and social conditions are just as important as a person's physical and psychological makeup and may have just as big an impact on their health.
- Treating the root cause or causes of a problem is more important than treating the obvious immediate symptoms. Treating only symptoms may simply cover up the real underlying problem and make it worse, so that it reappears later as something much more serious.
- Each person is an entirely original individual and cannot be treated in exactly the same way as every other person.
- Healing is quicker and more effective if the person takes central responsibility for his or her own health and has an active involvement in the healing process (but a good therapist will also recognize when someone needs to 'let go' and place themselves in the hands of another).
- Good health is a state of emotional, mental, spiritual and physical 'balance'. (Balance is fundamental to the

basic notion of health in natural therapy. Ill-health, say its exponents, is the result of being in a state of imbalance, or 'dis-ease'. The Chinese express this as the principle of *yin* and *yang*).

● There is a natural healing 'force' in the universe (what the Chinese call *qi* or *chi* – pronounced 'chee' – the Japanese *ki*, Indians *prana* and westerners *vis medicatrix naturae* or 'life force'). Anyone can 'tap into' or make use of this force and it is a natural health practitioner's skill to activate it in the patient or help the patient activate it in themselves.

It is natural therapists' belief in the Oriental ideas expressed particularly in the last two principles – and also often their use of those terms – that have caused so much controversy among so many doctors trained in the western scientific method. It is frequently the single most important reason they reject so much of it. (The reaction is probably understandable given the length of time they have spent in learning a very different system but the principles are there whether they like them or not. Moreover a blanket rejection of all therapies because of a refusal to accept, say, the concept of *qi* – 'life force' – stands the risk of throwing away something that may be beneficial simply because of a dislike of the trappings: the baby with the bathwater syndrome. The important thing is not to be put off just because some doctors get all huffy about it. They may be wrong!)

The essence of all natural therapies, however, is the same and returns very much to the earliest principles of medicine followed, practised and preached by the ancient healers of Greece and Egypt: that the best approach is the one that is the softest and gentlest, that avoids dangerous and traumatic procedures, that treats the patient as a 'whole' individual, and in which the patient takes an active part in his or her own recovery and health maintenance.

How do natural therapies treat heart disease?

Since they are neither synthetic drugs nor surgical techniques they operate by and large on a much more subtle level than the direct physical intervention favoured by conventional medicine. They can be seen as working basically in one of two ways (and sometimes a combination of both):

- treating your psychological condition by helping you to counter 'bad stress',
- treating your overall physical condition and increasing your level of 'well-being'.

In the treatment of heart disease they do this by:

- counteracting, reducing and eliminating psychological strain through relaxation
- helping you identify behaviour and habits that put you at risk
- clearing the arteries
- normalizing blood pressure
- stimulating the body's natural regenerative processes
- purifying the blood
- toning up tissues and organs.

That means they may work directly on one organ at the purely physical level or on all organs, tissues and blood at both physical and psychological levels. Results are seldom, therefore, immediate – although they can be – but the treatment is invariably gentle, always safe and frequently highly effective. In chapters 8 and 9 we will look at how, used in this way, they can help alleviate, reverse and even cure heart disease.

For how to find and choose a natural therapist see chapter 10.

CHAPTER 8

Treating your mind and emotions

Psychological therapies for your heart, blood and arteries

As we have seen in earlier chapters one of the most important risk factors – arguably even the single most important one – is mental and emotional strain. The word usually applied is 'stress' but the word on its own does not really tell us enough. In fact there is good stress and bad stress. Good stress is what keeps many people up and running. It can make us active, alert and ambitious. It can be a positive factor. Bad stress does not mean just extreme mental and emotional trauma. It may be the constant grind of being too pressurized, exhausted and angry too much of the time. Its damaging effect on the cells, tissues and organs of the body is well documented. In a word, it can be a killer.

Washington University stress experts Thomas Holmes and Richard Rahe showed 20 years ago that major life events – the top three were the death of a spouse, divorce and separation (job loss came out eighth, below marriage!) – are linked to illness in susceptible people by playing havoc with the body's biochemistry. But shock and pain are not as important as a cause of heart disease, or even a heart attack, as the long-term effects of suppressed hostility. People who live in a state of continual high pressure, easily aggravated and constantly irritable and unable to handle the hassles and inconveniences of daily life, are those most at risk of developing heart disease.

Their chances are highest of all if they have even one of the physical risk factors described in earlier chapters, and the chances multiply considerably for each extra one after that. But whatever the combination of factors – diet, lifestyle, stress, blood pressure and family trait – it does not happen overnight. It may take 20 or more years for heart disease to kill you this way – but kill you it will, as it already does every third man and every fourth woman, unless you do something about it.

There are natural treatments for heart disease which may help you manage and control the many forms of psychological dis-ease which cause this havoc. A central feature and aim of them all is to get you to relax and feel more 'at peace'. As Dr Ornish has proved, effective psychological treatment can halt the progress of heart disease and even reverse it by giving the body a chance to heal itself.

Again, the range of therapies and methods is many and varied, some proven and others not. They range from quite sophisticated approaches like those of hypnotherapy and psychotherapy to the very simple and charming, if perhaps fanciful, gem and crystal therapies. In between there is a wide spread of largely unrelated approaches from activity therapies, counselling, healing and homoeopathy to massage, meditation, visualization and yoga.

ACTIVITY THERAPIES

Therapies in this category are aimed mainly at releasing emotions locked up inside you such as anger, frustration, pain, despair and jealousy. Their purpose is to get you to work out your inner tensions and turmoils by involving you in some activity in which you are encouraged to express yourself outwardly. They include such approaches as art therapy, dance movement therapy, music and sound therapy, and group therapy. All need to be conducted under the guidance of an experienced therapist:

- **Art therapy** involves converting your emotions into colour, shape or form with any medium you like, be it paint, clay or chalk. You may be encouraged to throw paint violently against a large piece of paper or twist clay into whatever shapes you feel like, just to rid yourself of emotions that may be hurting you. Alternatively there may be no movement at all: the therapist may help you to express your inner feelings, violent or otherwise, simply by painting or drawing.
- **Dance movement therapy** can be practised on your own or in groups. The idea is to release tension by dancing in whatever way you want, freely and without inhibition.
- **Group or 'encounter' therapy** may involve sitting and talking your problems over with others or indulging in uninhibited exchanges that allow you to say things you perhaps would not normally have the courage to say but wish you could.
- **Music and sound therapy** is, again, a method of either making a noise yourself or responding to the noise of others. Hitting drums is one way of expressing anger in music and sound therapy, for example, but you may prefer simply to listen to the music of others played as loudly as possible.

COUNSELLING THERAPIES

As the name implies, counselling therapies generally encourage you to sit quietly and talk rationally about yourself and your problems to a trained and experienced listener or listeners who will help you find insights and see solutions for yourself. They include counselling, hypnotherapy and psychotherapy:

- **Counselling** is becoming such a well-organized, regulated and widespread therapy these days it is almost wrong to call it unconventional any longer. Nevertheless it is included because it is very clearly a safe and gentle treatment and extremely important in helping many people cope with major periods of stress and strain, whether a broken marriage, redundancy, debt or a sense of sexual inadequacy. In Britain and America it is increasingly common to find professional counsellors on the staff of health centres and clinics.

- **Hypnotherapy** (and hypnosis) is a very specific form of 'counselling', well supported by research, in which trained specialists, and they may be doctors as well as non-medical practitioners, aim to help you deal with unconscious or subconscious mental and emotional distress by placing you into a controlled hypnotic trance and helping you 'get in touch with' the cause or causes of the distress. Once the cause is revealed it may be easier to deal with it consciously through normal counselling or psychotherapy. Many hypnotherapists are also psychotherapists. Hypnotherapy is also a way of learning to relax deeply. The many 'subliminal' tapes now on the market use a form of hypnosis to aid relaxation.

- **Psychotherapy**, like counselling, is a method of getting you to understand and face up to psychological problems within yourself by talking them through with a trained listener. *It has nothing to do with psychiatry which is a purely medical discipline based largely on drug and surgical treatment of mental problems*. It can be done on either an individual basis or in a group. There is an enormous variety of psychological therapies available

STALK and SABRES: How not to die of a broken heart

British cardiologist Dr Peter Nixon believes there is a vital connection between physical effort and psychological break-down, which he has defined as 'the human function curve': when body and mind are required to do more than they can cope with they reach a point of exhaustion, followed by ill-health and finally complete breakdown. He has developed a programme for recovery from 'catastrophic stress' – severe stress leading to a physical breakdown – which he summarizes with the colourful acronyms STALK AND SABRES. If you are in crisis your first action is to STALK:

STOP everything and take time to re-evaluate what you are doing

THINK through the crisis and try and understand what it means

ACQUIRE information about possible treatment

LEADER: find someone to help you back to health

KNOWLEDGE: know about yourself and your relationship with the world.

Having decided your answers your next step is to perform SABRES:

SLEEP: sleep should be adequate, using hypnotherapy if necessary

AROUSAL should be modulated: do not get too excited or overwrought

BREATHING: avoid over-breathing (hyperventilation)

REST should be balanced out with

EFFORT: gentle to moderate exercise is probably beneficial

SELF-ESTEEM: the recovery of self-esteem through success.

Dr Nixon, who runs a stress-counselling clinic in London, believes a good therapist should offer support and guidance to someone in crisis rather than tell them what to do, and should avoid resort to drugs if at all possible. Ideally, the therapist should be part of a team with different skills who can pool their experience and resources on the patient's behalf.

– far more than there is room to list here – and they cover almost every type and style of approach, from the spiritually complex (such as psychosynthesis) to the down-to-earth (like laughter therapy). Research, particularly in Sweden, is showing that laughter therapy is extremely effective in releasing the sort of tension linked with aggressive 'type A' people and therefore very useful as part of a heart disease programme. Other psychological therapies you are likely to come across are co-counselling (or re-evaluation counselling), encounter therapy, gestalt therapy, humanistic psychology, psychodrama therapy, bioenergetics, Rogerian therapy, transpersonal psychology and transactional analysis. There are growing numbers of therapists who specialize in 'stress management' (such as Dr Peter Nixon, *see box opposite*) and often they will be in the best position to guide you towards the right psychological approach if they can't help you themselves.

RELAXATION THERAPIES

The very opposite of activity therapies, which deal mainly with violent emotion and frenzied activity, relaxation therapies aim to encourage a sense of deep inner peace and well-being by getting you to relax to such an extent you enter an almost dream-like state. They require conditions of quiet calm and the minimum of movement.

● **Meditation** is popularly seen as sitting in the famous 'lotus' position of the Indian yogis, legs crossed, hands together and eyes closed. But it need not be like this at all. Yoga and meditation are closely linked but it is possible to meditate lying in bed in the morning or sitting on a park bench provided nothing much else is going on around. The important thing is to listen to nothing but your own inner mind, the 'quiet centre' within yourself. 'Silent prayer' can be a form of meditation if you don't actually think but let the thoughts arrive of their own free will. Most of the many formal meditation methods have been imported into the West from the Orient, including the famous Transcendental Meditation (TM) and various yogas like hatha yoga, raja yoga and tantra yoga.

- **Autogenics** is a sort of western version of meditation, started in Canada, which combines some of the purposes of meditation with the techniques of auto-suggestion (made famous by the Frenchman Émile Coué with his *mantra*: 'Every day, in every way, I am getting better and better'). Often called 'passive concentration', it teaches six specific mental exercises to help you (actually your hypothalamus gland) switch off your normal 'fight or flight' responses and 'switch on the rest, relaxation and recreation system'.

- **Visualization** is a method often used in many meditative techniques positively to encourage your mind into a relaxed state by imagining any scene you like that is peaceful and restful. Counting sheep jumping over a fence to get to sleep is exactly the process. Therapeutically it has been used against cancer – patients are encouraged to imagine, for example, good white blood cells gobbling up or destroying harmful cells – and could be used in the same way in heart disease: you could imagine good cholesterol increasing and bad cholesterol reducing as (cider) vinegar pushing up oil in a jar.

- **Relaxing tapes and videos** are but the cheapest end of a blossoming market in mechanical aids for relaxation. Tapes and videos, of course, you can listen to or see at any time at home but some health centres offer them as part of a general relaxation programme, such as during 'floating' (floating inside a closed chamber of warm epsom-salts) or 'de-stressing' (lying in a special unit with your head outside, like a personal Turkish bath, so that different temperatures can be applied to your head and body: this apparently fools your mind into relaxing your body!). The British Holistic Medical Association publishes audio-tapes for relaxation as part of its *Tapes for Health* series.

- **Biofeedback** is a way of teaching yourself relaxation (and indeed meditation) by monitoring your relaxation responses with special equipment. For example, you could measure your brain-wave patterns (EEG) or blood pressure while relaxing and, depending on your responses, teach yourself to do more of what works and less of what doesn't. The idea is to help you confirm your mind in the ways it should work for best results for you.

PHYSICAL THERAPIES

It is no contradiction that physical activity can be the best form of psychological therapy. There is a strong link between mind and body and physical activity can be both a stimulant and relaxant with powerfully beneficial effects on the mind and hence to the body and back again. A number of therapies have, however, been developed which use physical activity as a form of meditation:

- **Yoga**, described further in the next chapter, is probably one of the best-known and most effective. It forms part of the programme created by Dean Ornish to cure heart disease naturally. Other versions extremely useful for heart patients because of their gentleness are the graceful *T'ai chi ch'uan* and the Oriental martial art *aikido*.
- **Massage**, again described further in chapter 9, is

another time-honoured way of achieving deep relaxation through physical therapy, this time at the hands of another (although massage can be self-administered). All the variations, like aromatherapy and reflexology (see chapter 9), apply just as much in the area of psychological benefit as in the physical – and, depending on the level of belief you apply to their medical claims, perhaps even more so.

- **Polarity therapy** is a highly unusual and original therapy which combines many elements of Oriental movement and meditation (yoga) and ayurveda (traditional Indian medicine) with western-style naturopathy, nutrition and healing. Founded this century by an Austrian doctor, Randolph Stone, who worked in both America and India, it claims to offer a complete physical and psychological healing system effective in almost any condition, including heart disease. Its systems have been worked out in great detail and it has some enthusiastic followers. But it suffers from both a lack of research and lack of practitioners.

SUBTLE ENERGY THERAPIES

Most of the therapies claiming to draw on paranormal, psychic or 'subtle' energies offer help for psychological disturbance but few produce much evidence for it. Many, like gem and crystal therapy, with their use of highly attractive gems and crystals, fall into the category of probably doing you good simply because they make you feel good – and that may well be justification enough: if it works don't knock it. The main therapies in this area for which there is actual evidence of benefit, however, are colour therapy, healing and homoeopathy:

- **Colour therapy**, although allegedly an ancient system, is in its infancy in the modern western world in many ways but there is still a respectable body of evidence that seems to show that colour can indeed affect the body as well as mood. For example, red has been shown to increase blood pressure and blue to reduce it. So there may be some benefit in consulting a therapist who will introduce you to colours you could surround yourself with to help your particular condition.

- **Healing, faith healing or spiritual healing**, claims to be able to effect both physical and psychological changes by the power of transmitted energy – either from God, the 'universal force' as some put it, or some other source. It may be applied by an individual or a group, and by direct hands-on touch or, as claimed by radionics, at a distance ('distant healing'). An Oriental method called *Qi Gong* (pronounced 'chee kung') is gaining a following in the West. There is not much to be said about healing except that it is the most researched 'natural method' after hypnosis and there is plenty of good evidence it works, believe it or not. Certainly if you feel it might help try it. It won't hurt.

- **Homoeopathy** is said to be one of the most powerfully effective therapies in many other conditions but does not have much to offer people with heart disease in any direct way. Like *flower remedies* (the most famous being the Bach Remedies and its 'Rescue Remedy'), it is of most help in addressing underlying patterns of behaviour and psychological conditions such as emotional trauma and stress. A skilled practitioner may be able to remove the causes of suppressed hostility or aggression, for example. Examples of the kind of homoeopathic remedies commonly given for heart-related problems are: as a general heart tonic *crataegus*, for breathlessness *arsenicum album*, for shock or bereavement *ignatia 30*, for depression under pressure *ac phos*, for strain and worry *argentum nitricum*, for 'stress' angina *cactus*. Homoeopathic remedies, like flower remedies, can be self-prescribed but it is best to consult an experienced practitioner for effective results.

Other options

Most of the information in this chapter has described psychological therapies of one kind or another, some you can do for yourself with a little initial help but most better tried through the services of an experienced practitioner or trainer. 'Type A' people *can* learn how not to be hostile, to become 'Type Bs' in other words. Cognitive and behavioural therapy or the 'rational-emotive' style of counselling may be effective ways of changing your personal reaction style. There is a growing body of opinion, however, that psychological therapies themselves – particularly those under the heading of 'counselling' such as humanistic and transpersonal psychology – may be less beneficial for someone with a heart problem than simply finding a good aromatherapist or reflexologist who is a good and intelligent listener as well as good with their hands. Many nurses and physiotherapists are also trained in such relaxation techniques these days. There is certainly a lot to be said for exercise rather than psychotherapy as a preferred treatment, particularly as far as men with 'hostile personalities' are concerned, and gentle *supervised* circuit training is well known to be highly effective as part of a healthy heart programme.

Summary

It is simply not possible to recommend a 'best buy' among each of the many therapies on offer. They might all be helpful or none at all. Your own individual needs and preferences are what counts and you cannot know

what might work until you try. There is no such thing as
a specialist in them all so the best way to find out is to
trust to intuition. That is, respond to whatever 'rings the
right bells', find out as much you need to know from the
sources listed at the end of this book and give one a try.
If you don't want to trust your own intuition find a practitioner who can help and guide you and follow their
advice. Details of how to find a reliable practitioner are
in chapter 10.

CHAPTER 9

Treating your body

Therapies for your heart, blood and arteries

The therapies described in this chapter all claim to improve your overall physical condition but particularly the condition of the organs and tissues of the circulatory system by working directly and indirectly on the immediate causes of heart disease. Their aim is to:

- clear blocked arteries
- rejuvenate the heart muscle and blood vessels, and
- clean and rejuvenate blood.

If effective they should return blood pressure to normal, remove symptoms of chest pain and breathlessness, and restore energy and strength. They range from natural 'medicines' like herbs, vitamins and minerals to physical therapies such as massage, hydrotherapy and yoga.

Nutritional supplements and herbs can be a powerful and direct way not only to prevent but also to treat heart disease naturally. There is evidence that correct treatment with the right nutrients – that is, vitamins, minerals, amino-acids and fatty acids – and herbs can help delay, prevent and even cure heart disease completely if taken regularly over a period of time. As a long-term measure regular supplements are as effective a prevention as a stress management programme, and the two approaches together can be a powerful shield against heart disease. But both nutrients and herbs, particularly those herbs known as 'adaptogens', can also be highly effective in dealing with established heart disease and are therefore well worth considering before synthetic drugs, and certainly before surgery.

Treatment using nutrients is called 'nutritional therapy' and with herbs 'herbal medicine' or 'phytotherapy'. So much success is being achieved with these methods that nutritional and herbal medicine could, together with stress management techniques, diet and exercise, become the number one treatment of choice for mild to moderate heart disease in the next century.

Nutritional therapy

Commonly known as 'food supplements' (because they are classified internationally as foods and not medicines, though there is some move in both North America and Europe to change this), the right nutrients in the right doses have the power to clear blocked arteries, improve blood, and rejuvenate blood vessels and heart muscle. Used in this intense way it is sometimes called 'super-nutritional therapy'.

Until recently many doctors poured scorn on the whole idea of taking supplements for health, insisting that a so-called 'balanced diet' provided all the nutrients needed. But a dramatic change of mind has been taking place, mainly because of the impact of research into antioxidants – nutrients which fight the causes of ageing and disease (see chapter 3).

In 1993 Professor Anthony Diplock, Britain's leading antioxidant researcher, confirmed what many eminent US researchers like Linus Pauling and Richard Passwater had been saying for years: that it was not possible to get sufficient antioxidant nutrients from food – and especially of the most important antioxidants vitamins A, C and E. Many researchers also insist that modern food production and preservation methods make most food, even fresh fruit and vegetables, so low in nutrients as to be nutritionally almost worthless.

Pioneer British nutritionist Dr Stephen Davies, who has often spoken out against what he calls 'the myth of the balanced diet', claimed at a conference in London in November 1993 that a ten-year survey of 65,000 people had shown that environmental pollution is exposing more people to levels of poisonous minerals the human body is not designed to deal with – notably lead, cadmium, aluminium and mercury. These levels not only increase with age (whereas levels of good minerals such as magnesium, zinc, chromium and selenium decrease) but they cancel out the effects of those nutrients we do get from food. His survey revealed that seven out of ten people were borderline or severely deficient in the vital B vitamins, for example. Extra supplementation is not only advisable, therefore, but essential.

Worldwide research is confirming almost by the month that regular intakes of antioxidant nutrients greatly increase resistance to heart disease and can add years to life. A major study of 13 European countries in 1993, for example, found that regular use of vitamins E, C and **beta carotene** (the natural vegetable source of vitamin A) almost doubled protection against heart disease. At the same time it found a low intake of the same vitamins exactly doubled your chance of getting heart disease and more than quadrupled your chance of stroke.

Experts make two important points about the prevention and treatment of heart disease by nutritional supplements:

- the longer and more regular the taking of supplements the better
- doses need to be much higher than the international recommended daily allowances (RDAs) to be of any value.

According to pioneer Dr Richard Passwater, for example, low levels of **vitamin E** are not only the single most important risk factor of heart disease but also a prime factor in angina. Regular supplementation with vitamin E not only protects against free radical damage but also reduces clotting in the blood and brings down blood pressure. But supplementation offers protection only if taken regularly for at least two years and shows maximum benefit after 15 years and more of regular use. He advises a therapeutic dose of between 400iu (international units) to 1200iu of vitamin E a day – 13 to 40 times the officially recommended amount in America!

The **vitamin C** story is another example. Animals, like plants, make their own vitamin C. Humans can't. One of the most important functions of vitamin C is to make collagen, vital for the manufacture of healthy human tissue including arteries. Vitamin C also stops cholesterol going 'rancid' (oxidizing), reduces the amount of dangerous lipoprotein-a in the blood and is instrumental in 'regenerating' vitamin E. Thus vitamin C deficiency can be a direct and major cause of arterial deterioration.

According to the world's leading expert on vitamin C, Linus Pauling, the body needs 12g (12,000mg) of vitamin C a day to function at optimal level in the modern world. Animals make this amount in their livers. Humans make none: the only vitamin C we get is from what we eat. The current international recommended daily amount (RDA) of vitamin C is just 60mg – *two hundred times below that required!* Even a diet high in fresh fruit and raw vegetables, the best natural source of vitamin C, would not provide anywhere near the huge amounts required says Professor Pauling. At 92, he takes 18g of vitamin C a day.

Fish oils are another set of nutrients effective against heart disease. Both Eskimo and Japanese peoples on a traditional diet have long been known to be relatively

Major antioxidants useful against heart disease

Nutrients	Action	Natural sources
Vitamin A (or as beta carotene)	Helps growth, sight and mucous membranes	Eggs, butter, liver, fish, carrots, peppers, beetroot
Vitamin C (ascorbic acid)	Regenerates vitamin E and connective tissue	Fresh fruit/*raw* vegetables
Vitamin E	Strong free radical fighter, triggered by selenium	Plant oils, fatty fish, leguminous fruits
Vitamin Q (Ubiqinone/ coenzyme Q10)	Responsible for energy production in cells	Lean meat
Vitamin B6 (pyridoxine)	Catalyst for other anti-oxidants (commonly deficient in elderly)	Cereal products, meat
Selenium	Protects against free radicals, triggers vit E	Fish, shellfish
Zinc	Helps attack free radicals	Liver, fish, eggs
Manganese	Another anti-free radical	Nuts, cereals, egg yolk

Note: Vitamins cannot work without minerals and amino acids to 'unlock' them.

Vitamins and heart disease

- In a 10-year study of 11,348 men and women between 1974 and 1984 at the University of California in Los Angeles (UCLA) survival rates from heart disease in those who took between five and ten times the RDA for vitamin C – that is, between 500-600mg a day – were 42 per cent better for men and 30 per cent better for women.
- Another study of 87,245 nurses between the ages of 34 and 59 showed a 40 per cent reduction in heart disease from regular supplementation with vitamins C and E.

heart disease-free. The reason? Their traditional diet is almost exclusively raw fish, and fish, particularly those found in colder waters such as salmon, herring and mackerel, are high in oils containing essential fatty acids. The main fatty acids effective against heart disease are *eicosapentaenoic acid* (EPA for short) and *gammalinoleic acid* (GLA). EPA is from the same class of fats – called omega 3 fatty acids – as those found in seed oils like sunflower, linseed and safflower, and vegetables. GLA, found in oil of the evening primrose, blackcurrant seeds and borage, is an omega 6 fatty acid. EPA is especially effective in bringing down blood fats as well as blood pressure and increasing the amount of good HDL cholesterol.

Another fat good for your heart is **lecithin**. Lecithin is a polyunsaturated fat and the principal component of HDL (good) cholesterol. Some 40 per cent of the brain is pure lecithin. It also happens to be a natural 'detergent' and is therefore one of the body's most powerful agents for dissolving arterial plaques. Regular supplementation with lecithin has shown dramatic reductions in such blockages. It also helps detoxify the liver and increases resistance to disease by supporting the work of the thymus gland. One of the best natural sources of lecithin, and protein generally, is eggs (but not too many: one recommendation is a maximum of four a week). Supplementary lecithin is usually bought as a grainy powder and sprinkled on food, but it is best to buy it vacuum-packed because it can go rancid.

Other **minerals** – apart from selenium, zinc and manganese (see table on page 116) – helpful against heart disease are magnesium, calcium, potassium, silica, molybdenum, iodine, boron and chromium. Silica (particularly high in bamboo) strengthens the walls of arteries and makes them more elastic. Magnesium, calcium (found in vegetables, dairy products, nuts and seeds) and potassium (found in fruit) can help lower blood pressure. Magnesium and calcium are a feature of hard water, which may be why less heart disease is found in hard water areas than soft. Magnesium (found particularly in almonds, sunflower and sesame seeds) is one of the most vital of all the minerals in heart disease. It is so important to the heart muscle and its arteries that in 1992 a UK trial supported the use of magnesium injected directly into the arteries to save heart attack victims from another attack.

Finally, certain of the 22 **amino acids** the body needs to function properly are considered extremely important in the prevention and treatment of heart disease. US nutritionist Dr Robert Erdmann recommends methionine, serine, carnitine, tryptophan and histidine, and Professor Pauling adds lysine. Dr Erdmann believes amino acids are the most important nutrients of all in the natural treatment of heart disease. Likening the causes of heart disease to a pebble that starts a landslide he claims amino acids have the ability unlike anything else to put the causes into 'rewind' so that, just like a rewound video of a landslide, everything goes back into its proper original place. Conventional drug treatments, on the other hand, he says, attack the end result but leave the debris where it is, causing blockage and chaos.

The most important aminos for heart disease are three of the eight so-called 'essential' amino acids (essential because the body can't make them):

● *Methionine* is a natural heavy metal 'chelator' (see 'chelation therapy' p. 117), promotes skin suppleness, helps reduce liver fat and protects the kidneys. As important, lack of it produces homocystine, a chemical 'sandpaper' that damages artery walls and thus encourages harmful deposits like lipoprotein-a (see chapter 4).

- *Tryptophan* is instrumental in maintaining healthy levels of the vital brain 'messenger' serotonin involved in controlling our behaviour patterns (see chapter 5). So it helps relieve all the types of behaviour leading to the build-up of 'bad stress' – and heart disease – such as anxiety, depression and insomnia. Research has shown as many as 15 per cent of the deaths caused by heart disease could be prevented by just this one amino acid.
- *Lysine*, according to Linus Pauling, is the most important of the amino acids for maintaining arterial and heart health. Present in large amounts in muscle tissues, it can reverse the hardening process in arteries, prevent the build-up of arterial deposits (plaques) and improve the tone of the heart muscle. Lysine (found mostly in wheatgerm, cottage cheese, chicken, wild game and pork) works closely with vitamin C and this has led Professor Pauling recently to declare that the two nutrients may be the single most important combination for heart health. He recommends a daily supplement of 1g of vitamin C and 3g of L-lysine, rising to 6g in severe cases of atherosclerosis.

Special note on supplements

Despite occasional scare-mongering in the media food supplements are so safe as to be almost fool-proof. They are not drugs any more than they are, strictly speaking, medicines. They are 'natural organic substances essential for life' (Dr Earl Mindell). Compared to drugs, with their hundreds of thousands of recorded deaths worldwide, supplements have an almost completely unblemished record. Only a few – the vitamins A, B_3 (niacin) and D and the minerals – have any toxicity at all, and then only if taken in *huge* doses. There is no evidence that food supplements do any harm even at high doses. That is some way, however, from saying that they guarantee to do you good. *Manufacturing quality is vital.*

Summary of supplements for heart disease

	Recommended daily amounts	
Vitamins	**Prevention**	**Treatment**
Vitamin A	20,000ius	20,000-40,000ius
as beta carotene	7,500ius	12,500-20,000ius
as retinol	7,500ius	7,500-15,000ius
Vitamin B3	30mg	50-250mg
Vitamin B6	25mg	50-100mg
Vitamin C	1000mg	2000-20,000mg
Vitamin E	200ius	400-1000ius
Biotin (vit H)	50mcg *(essential for vit C synthesis)*	
CoenzymeQ10 (vit Q)	40mg	60-150mg
Folic acid (vit M)	100mcg	200-450mcg
Minerals		
Calcium	350mg	350-800mg
Magnesium	175mg	175-500mg
Manganese	2.5mg	10-20mg
Selenium	100mcg	200-400mcg
Zinc	20mg	20-50mg
Amino acids		
Carnitine	250-1500mg	1500-3000mg
Histidine	250-1000mg	1000-3000mg
Lysine	3000mg	3000-6000mg
Methionine	250-1500mg	1000-3000mg
Serine	250-1000mg	1000-3000mg
Taurine	250-1000mg	6000mg
Tryptophan	*Currently banned in USA and UK*	
Fatty acids and fats		
EPA	180mg	300-3000mg
GLA	80-100mg	200-240mg
Lecithin	15000mg	45000mg

Dosage figures are given for guidance only. Treatment is best carried out under the guidance of an experienced practitioner.

Supplement ingredients should be of the right standard and purity and in the right combination. They should also be free of all additives, colourings and preservatives as well as allergen-free (no gluten, for example). Vegetarians should be aware that many capsules are made with gelatin and glycerine which comes from animals. Ground silica (similar to talcum powder) is also often used in tablets to bind ingredients together.

Unfortunately quality varies considerably, particularly in the USA where some of the worst 'capsule cowboys' are found. As a general rule, buyers should be wary of any supplement unless sold by one of the known reputable suppliers. Ask the shop or pharmacist when you buy what guarantees they have of the quality of the particular brand you want to buy. If they can't supply one don't buy but move to one they can guarantee.

Natural 'quick fix' treatments

Because natural therapies work slowly, over a period, there is an obvious lack of 'quick fix' emergency alternatives to surgery for heart disease but a few do exist that make this claim. The one with the most convincing track record to date is a form of super-nutritional therapy developed in America more than 30 years ago called 'Chelation (pronounced *Keylation*) therapy'.

Chelation therapy

This is a technique of slowly feeding a mixture of nutrients into the bloodstream by means of an overhead drip. The treatment takes about four hours and is usually given once or twice a week depending on the severity of the disease. For someone with severe arterial disease the recommended course is 20-30 intravenous infusions.

Technically chelation therapy is a process known as *chemo-endarterectomy* which means giving arteries a 'rebore' or 'decoke' by the use of chemicals. The three key ingredients *(see figure 8)* are an amino acid known as *ethylenediamine tetracetic acid* (EDTA), the anticoagulant heparin, and the trace element magnesium. Other ingredients are a variety of vitamins and minerals, including vitamins C, B1 and B5. EDTA is claimed to work by gradually dissolving arterial plaques so that they flush away through the kidneys in urine and most of the remaining nutrients have an antioxidant effect, encouraging regeneration of tissues and strengthening the body's immune system.

The film director Michael Winner, who became a highly publicized user of chelation therapy in the

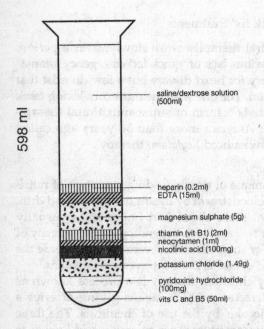

598 ml

saline/dextrose solution (500ml)

heparin (0.2ml)
EDTA (15ml)
magnesium sulphate (5g)
thiamin (vit B1) (2ml)
neocytamen (1ml)
nicotinic acid (100mg)
potassium chloride (1.49g)
pyridoxine hydrochloride (100mg)
vits C and B5 (50ml)

Figure 8 A typical Chelation Therapy infusion

autumn of 1993, described it as like 'flushing *Fairy Liquid* [a well-known UK washing up detergent] through your veins' and this is a reasonably accurate description of what happens – except all blood vessels are involved, especially arteries, and not just veins.

EDTA is in fact already well-known and accepted by doctors as a standard treatment for poisoning from heavy metals such as lead, mercury and cadmium but it is not accepted as a treatment for atheroma. The full-scale scientific trials needed for proof have not been done. Moreover some doctors are concerned that EDTA, originally developed in Germany to remove calcium stains from clothes and still used in food processing, is a toxic substance known to damage the kidneys in high doses.

In spite of the medical scepticism, the number of people treated worldwide is estimated to be approaching a million, more than half in North America where the number of doctors practising chelation is now over 300. But in some US states and in most of Canada it is banned. Opponents continue to claim EDTA not only removes calcium, making bones brittle, but also removes good minerals – like zinc and magnesium – from the body as well as bad.

Chelation's supporters, who include internationally known researchers such as Professor Pauling and Professor Emanuel Cheraskin, insist EDTA removes calcium from plaques not bones and that taking supplements replaces the beneficial minerals lost. They also insist its only known side-effects are good ones: improvements in hearing, sight and mental faculties.

On balance the evidence seems to be in favour of chelation. The lack of trials is a worry – in spite of claims the international drugs industry is trying to block them – and the need for regular supplementation to replace 'good' minerals lost during chelation is a serious caution.

How does EDTA chelation therapy work?

Doctors who practise EDTA chelation therapy believe it works by gradually dissolving calcium which is the binding 'cement' in arterial deposits (plaques). This then allows the body's natural defence mechanisms – assisted by diet, exercise, anti-stress and lifestyle counselling therapies – to take over the removal of the remaining debris hindering healthy blood flow.

Not only calcium deposits but also other harmful heavy metals such as lead, mercury and cadmium are 'clawed' out (the word 'chelation' is from the Greek *chele* meaning 'claw'). 'In fact the process is more one of binding than clawing: the EDTA binds harmful subtances to itself before flushing them away in the urine' is how the Arterial Health Foundation, the UK charity which supports chelation therapy, describes it.

Consultant Dr Wayne Perry, Britain's leading exponent of chelation for heart disease, claims 'the gist of chelation is anti heavy metal toxicity, anti clotting, anti lipid, anti calcium, anti cystine, anti free radical, anti arterial growth factor – thus opposing all the causes of atherosclerosis.'

Statistical evidence of trials in favour of chelation

In September 1993 the American *Journal for Advancement in Medicine* published a statistical review of all trials on chelation therapy published over the last 40 years, a so-called 'meta-analysis'. Carried out by two eminent Ohio researchers, the review identified 19 relevant papers covering a total of 22,765 patients. They found a 77 per cent success rate. This, the researchers concluded, shows statistically 'a high positive relationship between EDTA therapy and improved cardiovascular function'.

But these reservations aside chelation represents a much better and safer option than surgery for those with advanced or severe heart disease and is probably worth seeking out as a good intermediate measure in such cases.

Other 'quick-fix' techniques

Three other 'quick-fix' intravenous infusion techniques used in emergency 'natural' heart disease treatment are

---

CASE STUDIES

Brian Leigh, 60, property developer, of Sale, Cheshire (UK) had his first heart attack in 1977 at 43. A year later he underwent heart surgery and had five artery bypasses. Nine years later he had another heart attack and had another three artery bypasses. Within two years he began to feel unwell again and was thinking he might have to have further surgery when he heard about chelation. Over the next five months he received 20 infusions at the private Leigh Arterial Disease Clinic in Lancashire, England.

'It made a wonderful difference to my health. I experienced a tremendous improvement in my general well-being and vitality and I felt more alert and energetic. I could also concentrate better.'

He says the clinic encouraged him to change his diet and lifestyle: 'I now only eat things like fruit, salads, fresh vegetables, fish and granary bread - no fatty foods like cheeses and milk products.'

He still attends the clinic for 'top-ups' but claims the difference in his general health is 'startling'. He says he now swims up to 20 lengths of his local pool most weekdays and plays at least two games of golf every week. 'I am also back to working harder than ever.'

Simon Taylor, 32, marketing executive, of Stockton-on-Tees, Cleveland (UK) first felt chest pain and discomfort in 1987 at 25, a week after his wedding. A keen competitive athlete he was running about 60 miles a week and was 'fitter than ever'. Within two

---

months a cardiologist in London was recommending bypass surgery after an ECG and cardio-angiogram showed a main artery to his heart badly blocked. Surgery was planned for the following November.

In the following months his health deteriorated so badly that walking up two flights of stairs brought on chest pain. Then a chance conversation with marathon runner Leslie Watson put him in contact with the London chelation clinic. He started treatment and after about 16 infusions found 'things really began to look up'.

Today he trains twice a day five days a week, once on Fridays, and plays rugby on Saturdays. He lifts weights three times a week, runs one or two sprint sessions a week, plays 'at least' one game of squash a week and 'trys to get in two or three runs varying in distance from three to nearly five miles' every week.

He says he cannot train to the same sort of intensity he used to and he still gets some chest discomfort if he does not warm up properly – but 'compared to my level of fitness before chelation I am a totally different person'.

dimethyl sulphoxide (DMSO), hydrogen peroxide (H_2O_2) and ozone (O_3) therapy:

- **DMSO** is an avid free radical scavenger and is used in cases of severe arterial disease where blockages do not seem to respond to the supernutritional approach. But it is regarded as a dangerous technique by many and is practised hardly anywhere outside America.
- **H_2O_2** is better known as a bleach and disinfectant. Although a fast and efficient anti-viral agent, H_2O_2's anti-viral action is not only short-lived but it damages lipid membranes and accelerates free radical activity.

- **Ozone therapy** is a technique which increases the oxygen content of the blood in much the same way as hyperbaric oxygen therapy (see below) and with the same long-term dangers.

Special note

Specialists in this field all advise against taking EDTA, DMSO or H_2O_2 orally (by mouth), either in tablet or liquid form. EDTA is the less problematic of the three but studies have shown only 10-20 per cent absorption through the stomach wall and it is only effective if taken long-term as a preventive measure. There is some evidence that it is effective against depression taken this way, however.

Hyperbaric oxygen therapy

Another controversial 'natural' treatment for heart disease, hyperbaric oxygen therapy involves sitting inside a special sealed chamber at twice the normal atmospheric pressure while breathing in pure oxygen through a mask. This forces more oxygen into the bloodstream. Oxygen is a natural free radical 'scavenger' and the treatment is said to accelerate repair of heart and brain tissue as well as arteries. In Italy it is commonly used for stroke victims and elsewhere it may be used in the treatment of multiple sclerosis (MS). It is also increasingly popular with athletes who claim it improves performance by some 30 per cent and speeds recovery from injury by 40 per cent. A treatment session normally lasts from 1-2 hours. The main criticism of the technique is that it goes for short-term gain at long-term expense. Too much oxygen too quickly can produce intense energy in the body but accelerate oxidation and 'burn-out'.

Herbal medicine

For herbs to be used effectively in the treatment of serious heart disease it is vital that treatment should be carried out with the guidance and under the supervision of a qualified specialist. Herbal medicine is probably the earliest form of drug medicine known and herbs are powerful drugs. Indeed many modern drugs are directly derived from herbs. Foxglove, for example, has produced the powerful heart drug *digitalis* – but foxglove is a poisonous plant and is therefore extremely dangerous in untrained hands.

Doctors are generally not trained in herbal medicine but in Europe and North America there are specialists with a full and lengthy training in the subject. In the UK some practitioners undergo a specialist training as 'medical herbalists' or 'phytotherapists' but elsewhere it is more usual for the subject to be taught as part of a general training in natural medicine. Practitioners are then usually called 'naturopaths' or 'health practitioners' (*heilpraktikeren* in Germany).

There is surprising lack of good modern research into the efficacy of most herbs for the conditions they claim to help but most trained herbalists insist their use is part of a tradition handed down for centuries, and the proof they work is in the fact their reputation has survived for so long. Research is, however, picking up and studies, particularly in Europe, have already confirmed the benefits of such classic 'heart' plants as garlic, ginger, onion, hawthorn berry (crataegus), ginseng, pineapple (bromelain) and alfalfa. The following are some of the herbs claimed to be effective in treating specific diseases of the circulatory system (names in italics are said to be particularly effective):

Angina
Bromelain, garlic, *hawthorn berry* (or *crataegus*), lime blossom, lily of the valley and motherwort. (Long-term treatment with these herbs is said to completely remove all symptoms, but consult a qualified herbalist first.)

Atherosclerosis/Arteriosclerosis
Alfalfa, bromelain, bamboo, garlic, hawthorn berry, *lime blossom*, mistletoe and yarrow.

Diuretics (fluid releasers)
Broom, *dandelion*, lily of the valley and yarrow. (Dandelion contains high levels of essential potassium which is lost when synthetic diuretics are used.)

General heart tonics
Broom, bugleweed, figwort, hawthorn berries, *lily of the valley*, motherwort and night blooming cereus:
- *Broom* is a strong diuretic, getting rid of any buildup in body fluid from a weak heart as well as strengthening and normalizing the beat of the heart. It can increase blood pressure.
- *Bugleweed* reduces heart rate, increases heart strength and is a relaxant.
- *Figwort* increases the strength of heart contractions.
- *Hawthorn berry* is next in importance after lily of the valley. It strengthens heart muscle contractions and dilates (opens up) blood vessels.
- *Lily of the valley* is said to be highly effective against angina and the effects of an ageing heart as a result of clogged arteries. It is also a diuretic.
- *Motherwort* is a well-known heart strengthener and relaxer.
- *Night blooming cereus* has a similar action to lily of the valley and is particularly useful against irregularities in heart rhythm.

General tonics for the circulation
Broom, buckwheat, cayenne, dandelion, *ginger*, hawthorn berries, horse chestnut, lime blossom, mistletoe and yarrow.
- *Cayenne* and *ginger* stimulate circulation in the extremities.
- *Yarrow* is a diuretic.

Heart palpitations ('Nervous tachycardia')
Broom, bugleweed, hawthorn berries, mistletoe, *motherwort*, passion flower and valerian.

High blood pressure
Onion, buckwheat, cramp bark, *garlic*, hawthorn berries, lime blossom, mistletoe and yarrow.

Low blood pressure
Broom, gentian, ginseng, hawthorn berries, kola, *oats*, skullcap and wormwood.

Reducing blood fats (lipids)
Onion, *garlic* and ginger.

Stopping blood clotting
Bromelain, onion, garlic, *ginger*.

Tonics against anxiety and stress
Balm, *hops*, lime blossom, motherwort, pasque flowers, skullcap and valerian.

Varicose veins and ulcers
Buckwheat, cayenne, ginger, hawthorn berries, horsechestnut, prickly ash bark or berries.

Local swelling of ankles or legs
Dandelion or yarrow. For inflammation and pain use witch hazel, marigold, comfrey or hawthorn berries. For open wounds (ulcers) a compress of marigold, marshmallow and echinacea.

Phlebitis (blood clot in the leg)
Arnica, comfrey, hawthorn berries and marigold used as external lotions, compresses or poultices to relieve pain.

Except where described for external use (as lotions or compresses, for example) the above herbs are taken hot or cold as a 'tea'. But for best effect it is vital they are prepared in the right way. For example, high blood pressure can be treated with two parts hawthorn berries, lime blossom and yarrow to one part mistletoe drunk three times a day. But individual problems and symptoms may suggest adding cramp bark for tension, skullcap and valerian for anxiety and stress, or wood betony for headache. So consultation with an expert is really essential. An excellent source of further information for specific treatments by herbal medicines is *The New Holistic Herbal* by the herbalist David Hoffman (see Appendix B).

Herbs for the lymphatic system

The lymph glands and vessels are a much underappreciated part of the circulatory system. Their job is to help cleanse cells, tissues and organs by circulating body fluids back to the blood supply and supporting the body's immune system. Herbs which are claimed to help cleanse the lymphatic system are cleavers, echinacea, golden seal, marigold and poke root.

Naturopathy

Naturopathy is a term now in common use outside the UK, particularly in North America and Australia, to describe a range of 'natural therapies' from acupuncture to osteopathy offered by trained practitioners very much as an alternative or 'parallel' system to conventional medicine. In this approach they echo the system long established in Germany and parts of Europe where such practitioners are known as 'health practitioners' (*heilpraktikeren*). South Africa has a similar system but for local reasons its general practitioners are known as 'homoeopaths'. In Britain only a few hundred practitioners trained in this way exist and the trend, under government and medical pressure, is unfortunately towards a 'split therapy' approach.

Naturopathy is the modern version of what became known in the last century – and still is known to some – as 'Nature Cure', a fundamentalist approach to healing which believed absolutely in the body's power to heal itself given the right conditions: that is, the right diet, clean air and water, and plenty of exercise. The few Nature Cure (sometimes also called 'Natural Hygiene') practitioners who still exist – there are a handful in Britain and a number in continental Europe – support the use of relaxation and meditation but they do not believe in intervention of any other sort and would, for example, not even prescribe vitamins or herbs. Modern naturopaths have continued the basic philosophy but extended its practice.

The naturopathic approach is basically to get the body to heal itself by applying various techniques to correct physical, mental and emotional 'imbalances' (see chapter 7). In the case of heart disease, for example, these could consist of a combination of measures depending entirely on the strengths and weaknesses of the individual. For example, manipulation of the spine and muscles (osteopathy) might be used to correct stresses and strains caused by imbalances in the musculo-skeletal system, massage to relieve tension and relax tissues, acupuncture to reduce pain and improve 'vital energy', and hot and cold water compresses (hydrotherapy) to stimulate blood flow, and 'tone' blood and tissues. A naturopath would also be likely to recommend such techniques as colon and liver cleansing to improve the function of these vital organs, special diets, breathing and movement exercises (yoga) to improve mobility, circulation and oxygen intake and reduce stress, and cold baths to boost energy levels.

The important thing, again, is that although many of

these treatments can be done at home as self-help they are most effective if done under guidance as part of a programme geared to your specific needs prepared by the practitioner and yourself working carefully together.

Acupuncture   This is not (yet) a generally accepted form of treatment for heart disease in the West, but it is nevertheless commonly used in China in the treatment of angina, abnormal heart beat and high blood pressure. Studies in China and, recently, Scandanavia have shown an 80 per cent improvement in angina patients after acupuncture and up to 70 per cent improvement in *arrhythmias* (abnormal heart beats: palpitations, missed or irregular beats). Acupuncture with 'moxibustion' (a herb attached to the needle and allowed to smoulder to transfer heat) is the treatment for high blood pressure – although the Chinese do not see high blood pressure as a disease but as a symptom of a vital energy 'imbalance'. Acupuncture therefore treats symptoms such as dizziness and headache by claiming to stimulate the flow of *qi* (life force) around the body and removing any 'blocks'. Acupuncture is, however, well known and used in the West as a pain-killer – it releases pain-killing endorphins into the bloodstream – and this could be effective in relieving any painful effects of heart disease.

An increasingly popular form of treatment based on exactly the same principles but without the needles is *acupressure*. This literally uses hand or finger pressure (and sometimes feet or elbows) to achieve the same effect – and may even have been the original 'acu' system. Variations are *Shiatsu, Shen Tao, Jin Shen Do* (or *Jin Shin*) and *Do In*, which combines acupressure with exercise and breathing routines (see also 'Yoga' p. 134).

Colon cleansing   Colon cleansing (or 'colonic irrigation') is a technique of washing the colon (large intestine or gut) free of toxins (poisons) and the accumulated waste matter of years. Elderly people, especially women, can accumulate literally pounds of hardened material in their gut. The theory is that a clean colon can start to function more efficiently. Food should be digested and pass through the colon in about 20-24 hours but in people with 'caked' colons it can take more than 40 hours. In that time toxins build up and start to poison the body through the bloodstream. A prime cause of sluggish colons is too much refined and processed food with not enough fibre or 'roughage'. Practitioners claim that once the colon becomes lined with compacted waste – and it can come to resemble tyre rubber in colour and consistency in time! – the colon can no longer move to expel waste so well, and so it becomes trapped in a downward spiral of deterioration.

Colon cleansing – which is not the same as an enema – is a delicate and even risky technique and should only be done by a trained practitioner. Care has be taken to make sure that the equipment is sterile and that the right temperature and pressure is used to control the flow of water in the colon. Nausea may be felt during the procedure and extreme tiredness immediately afterwards. Careful eating, including supplementation with *acidophilus*, is necessary to re-introduce essential disease-fighting bacteria into the gut and prevent infection.

Hydrotherapy Always a central feature of the original 'Nature Cure' but ignored in recent years, hydrotherapy – water therapy – is making a strong comeback. Any form of therapy in, under or with water is hydrotherapy. With herbalism it is probably one of the oldest, most widespread and effective of all natural therapies. Hot springs, cold plunge pools and steam baths, for example, date back well before the Greeks and Romans and in every culture of the world. Health hydros, which were

once all the rage in Britain but now hardly exist anywhere, are commonplace in continental Europe where
whole complexes are given over to the benefits to be had
from simple water.

Almost any form of water therapy is beneficial in
heart disease. Swimming, for example, is an excellent
way to exercise and encourage mobility. But specific
forms of applied water therapy have also been shown to
improve the tone and efficiency of all the body's cells,
tissues and organs including the heart, blood vessels and
blood itself.

Cold water tips for heart health

- To improve heart and arterial function: pour cold water
  over your chest and back several times once a day for a
  month, followed by a few seconds dip in a cold bath or
  shower every morning.
- To improve circulation in the legs: pour cold water on the
  legs, from the knees down, twice a day morning and night.

You should do these exercises under the proper guidance
of a practitioner if you are elderly (the shock may do more
harm than good if you are not used to it). Some naturopaths
will prefer to treat you to the same effect themselves using
alternating towels soaked in hot and cold water. Among
other water treatments, available at most health hydros, are
such variants as sitz baths and Scottish douches (a hot and
cold jet spray).

Manipulation Techniques such as chiropractic,
osteopathy, cranial osteopathy and the Alexander
Technique do not claim to have a direct benefit in heart
disease but rather would hope to help indirectly. All are
concerned with problems that arise from 'bad posture',
the way of holding yourself which can lead to subtle and

unconscious but often powerful stresses and strains on your bones and muscles (the musculo-skeletal system). This can lead to illness of various sorts, including headaches and a greater susceptibility to stress, which can aggravate heart disease. Chiropractic (and its derivative McTimoney Chiropractic) and osteopathy focus on spinal irregularities for their main effect whereas cranial osteopathy (or cranio-sacral therapy), a refinement from osteopathy, and the Alexander Technique (AT) concentrate on the head and the way it sits on the shoulders. AT is a technique taught by a specialist (they prefer to call themselves 'teachers' rather than therapists) which, once learned, does not need a practitioner. The other three therapies have the potential to do considerable damage in the wrong hands and the services of a skilled practitioner is essential.

Massage   Another of the basic treatments as old as civilization now making a therapeutic comeback, massage is probably one of the most powerful ways known of relieving the sorts of physical and psychological tensions and stress that can accelerate heart disease. Probably because of its direct simplicity, as well as its effectiveness, it is being taken up worldwide in unprecedented numbers, including by professional healthcarers such as nurses who are using it increasingly in hospital and clinical situations.

Apart from pure massage itself – and there are any number of varieties, from the vigorous Swedish massage to altogether gentler almost touch-free ways of some 'therapeutic massage' such as polarity therapy and therapeutic touch – there are its highly popular derivatives aromatherapy and reflexology.

Aromatherapy This uses a wide range of scented concentrates from plants which it claims have certain therapeutic effects if massaged into the body with oil. (Strictly speaking, aromatherapy is 'smell therapy' and its specialists point out that the scents can be used in many other ways – by being inhaled, vaporized, put into a hot compress or even gargled – but it is its use in massage which is most popular.) For example, aromatherapists claim that grapefruit oil is useful against arterial deposits, marjoram and ylang-ylang against high blood pressure, and rose against emotional trauma. But just as with supplements, the quality of concentrates varies enormously, and though there is a growing body of evidence which seems to show that aromatherapy is effective in achieving the results it claims there is nothing like the same certainty with the quality of some of the oils now flooding the market. You probably get what you pay for but the safest bet, and by far the most pleasurable, is to find a good and knowledgeable aromatherapist to help you.

Reflexology This is another therapy, like aromatherapy, whose popularity has grown enormously due to its simple and direct hands-on approach. There is much discussion about whether its central claim is correct – that using the same sort of 'energy pathways' theory as in traditional Chinese medicine it can create physical changes through pressure on special 'reflex' points in the feet and hands – but its use simply as a highly effective relaxant probably justifies its existance. Among variants are:

- *Zone therapy*
- *The Metamorphic Technique*, and
- *Vacuflex therapy*, a particularly interesting high-tech

version which uses vacuum pressure and rubber pads reminiscent of Oriental 'cupping' for quicker results.

Reflexology can be used as self-help (except Vacuflex) but a competent and knowledgeable therapist is better.

Special diets Some naturopaths may recommend a so-called 'mono-diet' for heart disease, which involves eating just one type of food for several days. Two of the best known are the 'Grape Cure' and the 'Rice Diet'. The Grape Cure, eating nothing but grapes (up to 3kg a day, with water, grape or apple juice to drink), is said to bring down blood pressure, tone up the heart and remove excess fluid. The Rice Diet (eating around 300g of boiled or steamed rice every day with a little to drink and some fruit) is supposed to be useful against obesity and heart disorder generally. As with fasting (chapter 5), it is not a good idea to go on a special diet of this severity without supervision. Another special diet is the Pritkin Diet, a low-everything diet (low fat, low carbohydrate, low oil and so on) used with success in Dean Ornish's famous 'Lifestyle Heart Trial' in California.

Yoga Another ancient system, yoga is not intended primarily as a therapeutic technique at all. The word is ancient Indian for 'union' (the English word 'yoke' comes from it) and at its highest level it is a method of achieving union with the Divine or God through a special way of life – of which exercises and special breathing techniques are a central part. Ayurvedic medicine (traditional Indian medicine) is also an offshoot. At a basic level yoga exercises (for example, the exercise 'The Cat', *figure 9*, or the more involved 'Salute to the Sun') and yoga breathing are simple physical and mental practices that are highly effective ways of improving mobility, suppleness, blood

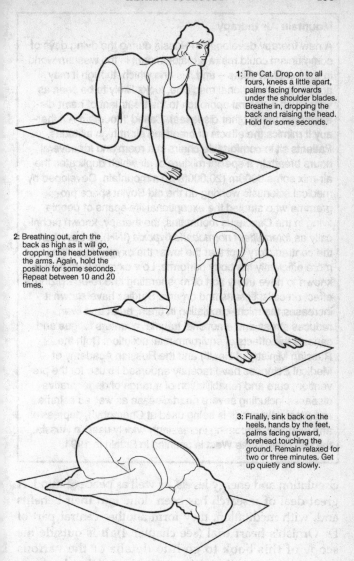

1: The Cat. Drop on to all fours, knees a little apart, palms facing forwards under the shoulder blades. Breathe in, dropping the back and raising the head. Hold for some seconds.

2: Breathing out, arch the back as high as it will go, dropping the head between the arms. Again, hold the position for some seconds. Repeat between 10 and 20 times.

3: Finally, sink back on the heels, hands by the feet, palms facing upward, forehead touching the ground. Remain relaxed for two or three minutes. Get up quietly and slowly.

Figure 9 Simple yoga exercise: 'The Cat'

Mountain Air therapy

A new therapy developed in Russia during the dying days of communism could make a major impact in the western world in the next few years – and it is one which, though it may appeal to conventional medicine, looks likely to be seen as very much a natural approach to the treatment of heart disease (and many other diseases). Called 'Mountain Air' therapy it mimics the effects of breathing air at high altitudes. Patients sit in comfortable chairs in a room and for several hours breath in a special mixture of air which duplicates the air-mix some 6000m (20,000ft) up a mountain. Developed by medical scientists working on the old Soviet space programme who studied the exceptional life-spans of people living in the Caucasus mountains, the therapy, known technically as *intermittent normobaric hypoxia* (INH), is based on the contradictory fact that the lower the oxygen level the more efficiently the body performs. Low oxygen (hypoxia) is known to have every sort of regenerating and re-energizing effect on cells, tissues and organs. Studies have shown it increases the micro-circulation in brain, heart and liver, reduces stress and emotional trauma, counters fatigue and cancels the effects of environmental pollution. Both the Russian Ministry of Health and the Russian Academy of Medical Sciences have recently endorsed its use for the prevention, cure and rehabilitation of a range of degenerative diseases including severe heart disease as well as asthma, radiation sickness (it is being used at Chernobyl), depression and allergies. Becoming increasingly widely used in Russia, the first clinic in the West is opening in Britain in 1994.

---

circulation and energy levels, as well as peace of mind. A great deal of research has been done into their benefits and, with meditation, they form another central part of Dr Ornish's heart trial (see chapter 4). It is outside the scope of this book to go into details of the various techniques in yoga but there are many excellent books on the market which do. (*The Natural Way With Asthma,* another in this same series by Element Books, contains some breathing and movement exercises that can also be helpful in improving heart health.)

'Energy' therapies

There are a host of so-called 'energy therapies' that claim to draw on some subtle healing 'power' or 'life force' for their effect. They include gem and crystal therapy (and its modern extension electro-crystal therapy) and radionics. Radionics, for example, claims to be able to 'reconstitute' organs as good as new by a type of metaphysical or psychic reprogramming using a piece of equipment which 'channels' subtle energies. But there is no hard evidence for this – and indeed no evidence that any energy therapies are effective in the physical treatment of heart disease. Anyone who wishes to try any of these approaches should do so in the knowledge that they are certain to do you no harm and may help but we simply can't be sure. Belief or faith in both the therapy and therapist seems to be as important as anything in their success and with the right person there may well be benefit.

Summary

The message of this chapter, and of the book as a whole, is to find the right practitioner. It cannot be said or emphasized enough that the therapist is often more important than the therapy. Good support from a practitioner, and the chance to unload and unwind, are always a help. So for the best advice on natural physical treatments for heart disease consult *either* an enlightened doctor *or*, and possibly as well as, the best naturopath and/or nutritionist you can find. We'll look at how to find and choose the right therapist next.

ın

How to find and choose a natural therapist

Tips and guidelines for finding reliable help

It is unfortunately not as easy as it should be to find the right therapist. Although natural medicine is enjoying a boom and everyone seems to want to use it, diversity, competition between groups and duplication within therapies has made the task a difficult one in most countries in which natural medicine is growing in popularity. It is the main purpose of *The Natural Way* series to help you find the right gentle therapy for your condition – but finding the right practitioner or therapist is in some ways the harder task.

The best answer is almost always personal recommendation, and this applies as much to doctors as nonmedical practitioners. Go to someone a friend or someone you trust has recommended. As a rule of thumb it cannot be bettered. But if you still cannot get a good recommendation what next? There are several options:

● Go to your local doctor's clinic or health centre and ask their advice. It may take some courage and you may not get a sympathetic response but it is worth a try, and you may get a pleasant surprise: you may find they have the very person you need – either someone who helps at the clinic or to whom patients are referred (which means, in countries with a state health service, possibly free treatment).

- Your nearest natural health centre may be able to help, or even a natural health practitioner who you know is not the right person for you but who may be prepared to recommend someone else who may be. This way is not as good as personal recommendation but therapists who specialize in natural therapy tend to know who else is at work in their area and, more important, who is any good. You can get the names of centres and individual practitioners to approach from healthfood shops, *Yellow Pages* or local listings in newspapers, magazines, citizen advice and information centres and libraries. If you are into computers and have a modem, computer networks have lists. A particularly good bet is a natural health centre in your area which has several practitioners with different skills working at it. The better centres have a system where a patient contacting them for help will be offered a consultation in which his or her case is considered by a panel of practitioners and a therapy or therapies and a therapist or therapists recommended. Such an approach is still in its infancy, though, so it may be hard to find.

- Failing a local recommendation or the availability of an enlightened group practice, the next step is to contact any of the national therapy 'umbrella' organizations and ask for their list(s) of registered organizations or practitioners. Their addresses are listed in Appendix A. They may charge for their lists (especially for postage and packing) and insist you select not only which therapy but also, because there is still no one recognized organization for each therapy in many countries, which particular organization you want a members' list of. If you can afford it ask for the lot.

> **10 ways of finding a therapist**
> - word-of-mouth (usually the best method)
> - your local family medical centres
> - your local natural health centres
> - your local healthfood shops
> - health farms and beauty treatment centres
> - local patient support groups
> - national therapy organizations (but see below)
> - computer networks (you need a 'modem')
> - public libraries and information centres
> - local *Yellow Pages*, newspapers and magazines

Checking professional organizations

Whether or not you have found a therapist straight away it is still a good idea to check on their professional background. This becomes almost essential if you are picking a name from a list rather than following a recommendation from a friend. Just because a therapist belongs to an organization doesn't mean he or she comes with a guarantee. Some organizations do no more vetting of their members than making sure they've paid their membership fees.

The first thing to do is to check the status of the individual associations or professional organizations whose names you have got. A good association will publish the information clearly and simply in the same booklet as its members list. Few seem to, however, and so you may have to ring them up or write to them. The following are the sort of questions you should try and get answered:

- When was the association founded? (Groups spring up all the time and you may find it useful to know if they have been going 50 years or started yesterday.)
- How many members does it have? (Size will give you

a good idea of its public acceptance and genuine aims.)

- Is it a charity or educational trust – with a formal constitution, an elected committee and published accounts – or is it a private limited company? (Private companies can be secretive and self-serving.)
- Is it part of a larger network of professional organizations? (Groups that go their own way are on balance more suspect than those who 'join in'.)
- Does the association have a code of ethics, complaints mechanism and disciplinary procedures? If so, what are they?
- Is the association linked to one particular school or college? (One that is may have no independent assessment of its membership; the head of the association may also be head of the college.)
- What are the criteria for membership? (If it is graduation from one particular school or college the same problem arises as above.)
- Are members covered by professional indemnity insurance against accident and malpractice?

Checking training and qualifications

Next you may want to try and satisfy yourself about their training and qualifications. A good listing will, again, describe the qualifications and say what the initials after every member's name mean. Yet again, few seem to. So it's a case of ringing or writing to find out. Questions to ask are the following:

- How long is the training?
- Is it full-time or part-time?
- Does it include seeing patients under supervision?
- Is the qualification recognized?
- If so, by whom?

The British Medical Association's opinon

In its long-awaited second report into the practice of natural medicine in Britain, published in June 1993, the British Medical Association recommended that anyone seeking the help of a non-conventional therapist – doctor or patient – should ask the following questions:

- Is the therapist registered with a professional organization?
- Does the professional organization have
  a public register?
  a code of practice?
  an effective disciplinary procedure and sanction?
  a complaints mechanism?
- What qualification does the therapist hold?
- What training was involved in getting the qualification(s)?
- How many years has the therapist been practising?
- Is the therapist covered by professional indemnity insurance?

The BMA said that although it would like to see natural therapies regulated by law, with a single regulating body for each therapy, it did not think that all therapies needed regulating. For the majority, it said, 'the adoption of a code of practice, training structures and voluntary registration would be sufficient.'

Complementary Medicine: New Approaches to Good Practice (Oxford University Press, 1993).

Making the choice

The final choice is a matter of using a combination of common sense and intuition and giving someone a try. But do not hesitate to double-check with them when you see them that the information in the listing agrees with what they tell you – nor to cancel an appointment (give at least 24 hours notice if you can) or to walk out if you do not like anything about the person, the place or the treatment. The important advice at all times is to ask questions, as many as you need to, and use your intuition. Never forget: it is your body and mind!

What is it like seeing a natural therapist

In a word, different. But it is also very natural. Since most therapists, even in those countries with state health systems, still work mainly privately there is no established uniform or common outlook. Though they may all share more or less a belief in the principles outlined in chapter 7 you are liable to come across individuals as different as chalk from cheese, representing all walks of life, from the rich to the poor, the politically left to the politically right. That means you will come across as much variety in dress, thinking and behaviour as there are fashions, from the elegant and formal to the positively informal and 'woolly-haired' (though, for image reasons, many now wear a white coat to look more like a doctor!).

Equally, you will find their premises very different – reflecting their attitudes to their work and the world. Some will present a 'brass plaque' image, working in a clinic or room away from home with receptionist and brisk efficiency, while others will see you in their living room surrounded by pot plants and domestic clutter. Remember, though, image may be some indication of status but it is little guarantee of ability. You are as likely to find a therapist of quality working from home as one in a formal clinic.

There are some characteristics, however, probably the most important ones, you will find common to all natural therapists. They will:

- Give you far more time than you are used to with a family doctor. An initial consultation will rarely last less than an hour, and often longer. During it they will ask you all about yourself so they can form a proper understanding of what makes you tick and what may be the fundamental cause(s) of your problem.

- Charge you for their time and for any remedies they prescribe, which they may well sell you themselves from their own stocks. But many therapists offer reduced fees, and even waive fees altogether, for deserving cases or for people who genuinely cannot afford it.

Sensible precautions

- Though most practitioners practice for fees no ethical person will ask for fees in advance of treatment unless for special tests or medicines, but even this is unusual. If you are asked for 'down payments' of any sort ask exactly what for and if you don't like the reasons refuse to pay.
- Be sceptical of anyone who 'guarantees' you a cure. No one (not even doctors) can.
- Be very wary of stopping drugs prescribed by your family doctor on the therapist's insistence without first talking things over with your doctor. Non-medical therapists know little about pharmaceutical drugs and there may be danger to yourself if you stop suddenly or without preparation.
- If you are female feel free to have someone with you if you need to undress and if being accompanied makes you feel more comfortable. No ethical therapist will refuse such a request, and if they do have nothing more to do with them.

What to do if things go wrong

The most important thing to decide is whether you think the therapist has done their absolute best to get you better without hurting or harming you in any way. Failure to cure you is not an offence (the truth is it is probably as much as disappointment to the therapist as it is to you) but failure to take proper care and treat you with professional respect is. If this should happen to you, and you feel it is as the result of behaviour which you regard as either incompetent or unethical, you could consider the following actions:

- If you feel the therapist was doing their best to help – and most obviously try to – but simply wasn't good enough it might be as well, for the safety of future patients as much as for the therapist's sake, to talk the problem over with him or her first. They may be oblivious of their shortcomings and be not only grateful for your constructive honesty but see a way to make amends and help you further. But if the situation is more serious than this then you have no option but either to turn your back on the whole episode or take action. If you decide to take further action the courses open to you are:

- Report them to their professional association or society if they have one. (Don't expect this to lead to dramatic changes however. Because unconventional medicine still belongs in many ways to an unestablished, and even sometimes anti-establishment, subculture – it has been called 'the folk medicine of the masses' – it exists in many countries still in a sort of unregulated limbo world in which pretty well anything goes and there are few official controls. This can have its advantages of course: the better and more original practitioners can experiment and change direction at will in a way they wouldn't be allowed to do if they were tied up in rules and regulations as doctors are. But it also means there is little or no professional comeback if they don't behave in a way you like or think they should. Even if they belong to a professional organization – and, in Britain at least, no practitioner who is not medically trained has to belong to any organization – those organizations have little or no real power to do anything to a member who breaks the rules. In Britain if they expel someone that person is still free to practice under existing common law provided they don't break any civil or criminal law.)

- Tell anyone and everyone you come across about your experience, especially the person who recommended the therapist if this applies, and tell the therapist himself or herself you are doing so (but make sure you are telling the truth: deliberately spreading lies which damages someone's reputation and livelihood is a criminal offence). Practitioners who get themselves a bad reputation are quickly out of business – and rightly so – and so to that extent, at least, they are under pressure to behave professionally, and they know it. Ultimately that is your only guarantee. But it is also the best guarantee.

- In the very worst case, which is always possible though rare, you can resort to the civil or criminal law – that is, you can sue or bring a charge for assault – either through a lawyer or by going direct to the police. Alternatively citizens rights or advice bureaux may be able to help.

Summary

The reality is that although the opportunity is there, resulting in the occasional tabloid newspaper headline, there are few real crooks or charlatans in natural therapy. Despite the myth, there is little real money in it unless the therapist is very busy – and if he or she is the chances are high it is because he or she is good. In fact you are just as likely to find bad practitioners in orthodox medicine and among the ranks of the so-called 'qualified' as among those who work quietly alone at home with no formal training at all. No one can know everything and no one qualified in anything, including medicine, has to get 100 per cent in their exams to be able to practice. Perfection is an ideal not a reality and to err is human.

It is very much for this reason that taking control of your own health is perhaps the single most important lesson underlying the series of books of which this is part. For taking control means taking responsibility for the choices you make, and taking responsibility for choices we now know to be one of the most significant factors in successful treatment, whether of yourself or through the intermediate services of a therapist. No one else but you can decide on a practitioner and no one else but you should decide if that practitioner is any good or not, whether they are a conventional doctor or a natural therapist, or both. You will know very easily, and probably very quickly, if they are any good by the way you feel about them and their therapy and by whether or not you get any better.

If you are not happy about them or your progress the decision is yours whether to stay or move on – and continue moving until you find the right therapist for you. But do not despair if you don't find the right person first time, and above all never give up hope. There is almost bound to be the right person for you somewhere and your determination to get well is the best resource you have for finding them.

Above all, bear in mind that many people who have taken this route before you have not only been helped beyond their most optimistic dreams but have also found a close and trusted helper who they, and their family, can always turn to in times of trouble – and who may even become a friend for life.

APPENDIX A

Useful organizations

The following listing of organizations is for information only and does not imply any endorsement, nor do the organizations listed necessarily agree with the views expressed in this book.

INTERNATIONAL

International Federation of Practitioners of Natural Therapeutics
46 Pulens Crescent
Sheet
Petersfield
Hampshire GU31 4DH, UK.
Tel 0730 266790
Fax 0730 260058

International Society & Federation of Cardiology
34 Rue de l'Athenee
PO Box 117
CH-1211 Geneva 12
Switzerland.
Tel 22 347 6755
Fax 22 347 1028
Formed in 1978 to coordinate the activities of national and regional heart research and education bodies. Currently 64 countries represented.

AUSTRALASIA

Australian Natural Therapists Association
PO Box 308
Melrose Park

South Australia 5039.
Tel 8297 9533
Fax 8297 0003

Australian Traditional Medicine Society
PO Box 442 *or*
Suite 3, First Floor
120 Blaxland Road
Ryde
New South Wales 2112.
Tel 2808 2825
Fax 2809 7570

National Heart Foundation of Australia
PO Box 2
Woden
ACT 2606, Australia.
Tel 6 282 2144
Fax 6 282 5147

National Heart Foundation of New Zealand
PO Box 17-160 *or*
17 Great South Road
Newmarket
Greenlane
Auckland 5, New Zealand.
Tel 9 524 6005
Fax 9 524 7854

New Zealand Natural Health
Practitioners Accreditation
Board
PO Box 37-491
Auckland, New Zealand.
Tel 9 625 9966
*Supported by 15 therapy
organizations.*

NORTH AMERICA

**American Academy of Medical
Preventics**
6151 West Century Boulevard,
Suite 1114
Los Angeles
California 90045, USA.
Tel 213 645 5350

**American Association of
Naturopathic Physicians**
2800 East Madison Street
Suite 200
Seattle
Washington 98112, USA
or
PO Box 20386
Seattle
Washington 98102, USA.
Tel 206 323 7610
Fax 206 323 7612

**American College for
Advancement in Medicine**
23121 Verdugo Drive
Suite 204
Laguna Hills
California 92653, USA.
Tel 714 583 7666
Fax 714 455 9679
*Promotes, monitors and controls the
practice of chelation therapy
worldwide.*

**Association for Cardiovascular
Therapies**
PO Box 706
Bloomfield
Conn 06002, USA
Tel 203 724 0081
*A national non-profit organization
founded in 1978 by heart patients to
promote 'natural' therapies in the
prevention and treatment of heart
disease, particularly chelation
therapy.*

American Heart Association
7272 Greenville Avenue
Dallas
Texas 75231, USA.
Tel 214 373 6300
Fax 214 706 1341

**American Holistic Medical
Association**
4101 Lake Boone Trail, Suite 201
Raleigh
North Carolina 27607, USA.
Tel 919 787 5146
Fax 919 787 4916

**Canadian Cardiovascular
Society**
360 Victoria Avenue, Room 401
Westmount
Quebec H3Z 2N4, Canada.
Tel 514 482 3407
Fax 514 482 6574

**Canadian Holistic Medical
Association**
700 Bay Street
PO Box 101, Suite 604
Toronto
Ontario M5G 1Z6, Canada.
Tel 416 599 0447

**Heart and Stroke Foundation of
Canada**
360 George Street, Suite 280
Ottawa
Ontario K1N 9B2, Canada.
Tel 613 237 4361
Fax 613 234 3278

**National Heartsavers
Association**
4601 South 76th Street
Omaha
Nebraska 68127, USA.
Tel 402 339 3813

**Solgar Nutritional Research
Center**
Ocean Pines
11017 Manklin Meadows Lane
Berlin
Maryland 21811, USA.
Tel 410 641 7411

**Preventive Medicine Research
Institute**
900 Bridgeway, Suite 2
Sausalito
California 94965, USA.
Tel 415 332 2525
Information freephone line
800 328 3738

SOUTHERN AFRICA

**South African Homoeopaths,
Chiropractors & Allied
Professions Board**
PO Box 17055
0027 Gooenkloof
South Africa
Tel 2712 466 455

**UK
British Complementary
Medicine Association**
St Charles Hospital
Exmoor Street
London W10 6DZ.
Tel 081-964 1205
Fax 081-964 1207

**Council for Complementary &
Alternative Medicine**
179 Gloucester Place
London NW1 6DX.
(Tel 071-724 9103
Fax 071-724 5330

**Institute for Complementary
Medicine**
PO Box 194
London SE16 1QZ.
Tel 0721-237 5165
Fax 0712-237 5175

British Diabetic Association
10 Queen Street
London W1M 0BD.
Tel 071-323 1531
Fax 071-636 3096

**British Holistic Medical
Association**
179 Gloucester Place
London NW1 6DX.
Tel 071-262 5299

Health Education Authority
Hamilton House
Mabledon Place
London WC1H 9TX.
Tel 071-383 3833
Fax 071-387 0550

UK HEART CHARITIES
A total of 138 charities whose work relates to heart disease and its sufferers are registered in the UK with the Charity Commission in London. The commission holds a central register and database and will check any charity for you (ring 071-210 4405/ 4533/4685). The following are the main organizations in the field:

Arterial Health Foundation
57A Wimpole Street
London W1M 7DF.
Tel/fax 071-935 6604
Britain's newest and smallest heart charity (founded 1991), specializing in research into and education of what it calls 'safe and gentle alternatives' for the treatment of heart disease, particularly chelation and antioxidant therapies.

British Heart Foundation
14 Fitzhardinge Street
London W1H 4DH.
Tel 071-935 0185
Fax 071-486 1273
Britain's largest private heart and arterial disease research organization and largest heart research charity, with an annual income of over £31 million (1992).

Family Heart Association
Wesley House
7 High Street
Kidlington
Oxford OX5 2DH.
Tel 08675 70292
Full name the Familial Hypercholesterolaemia and Familial Hyperlipidaemia Association, the charity is geared towards people with a genetic tendency towards high cholesterol and lipid levels and aims to help them lower those levels as well as identify others at high risk by promoting cholesterol screening and healthy eating.

The Stroke Association
CHSA House
Whitecross Street
London EC1Y 8JJ.
Tel 071-490 7999
Fax 071-490 2686
Formerly the Chest, Heart and Stroke Association (established in 1899), the only national charity concentrating on trying to reduce the number of people suffering from strokes through research, prevention and direct help for sufferers and their families.

Yoga for Health Foundation
Ickwell Bury
Biggleswade
Bedfordshire SG18 9EF
Tel 0767 627271

UK PATIENT SUPPORT GROUPS

British Cardiac Patients Association (The Zipper Club)
6 Rampton End
Willingham
Cambridge CB4 5JB.
Tel 0954 260731
For the help and support of people who have had by-pass surgery.

APPENDIX B

Useful further reading

Acupuncture, George Lewith (Thorsons, UK, 1982)

Conquering Heart Disease, Richard Brown (Arterial Health Foundation, UK, 1990)

Dr Dean Ornish's Program for Reversing Heart Disease, Dean Ornish (Random House, USA, 1990)

Encyclopaedia of Natural Medicine, Michael Murray & Joseph Pizzorno (Macdonald Optima, UK, 1990)

Forty Something Forever: A Consumer's Guide to Chelation Therapy and Other Heartsavers, Arline and Harold Brecher (Healthsavers Press, USA, 1992)

Healing and the Mind, Bill Moyers (Doubleday, USA, 1993)

Healing the Heart, Elizabeth Wilde McCormick (Optima, UK, 1992)

How to Live Longer and Feel Better, Linus Pauling (W H Freeman, USA, 1986)

Mind-Body Medicine: How to Use Your Mind for Better Health, ed Daniel Goleman and Joel Gurin (Consumer Reports Books, USA, 1993)

Mind, Stress and Health, Richard Totman (Souvenir Press, UK, 1990)

Nutritional Medicine, Stephen Davies & Alan Stewart (Pan Books, UK, 1987)

Reader's Digest Family Guide to Alternative Medicine, ed Dr Patrick Pietroni (The Reader's Digest Association, UK, 1991)

The Alternative Health Guide, Brian Inglis & Ruth West (Michael Joseph, UK, 1983)

The Alternative Dictionary of Symptoms and Cures, Caroline Shreeve (Century Hutchinson, UK, 1986)

The Amino Revolution, Robert Erdmann & Meirion Jones (Century, UK, 1987)

The Complete Yoga Course, Howard Kent (Headline Press, UK, 1993)

The New Holistic Herbal, David Hoffman (The Findhorn Press/Element Books, UK, 1990)

The Vitamin Bible, Earl Mindell (Arlington Books, UK, 1982)

Will to be Well, Neville Hodgkinson (Hutchinson, UK, 1984)

Index